Spoken/Unspoken

Hidden mechanics of the patient-doctor relationship

Selected posts from the *Illusions of Autonomy* blog

By Philip Berry MD MRCP

All illustrations are by the author

By the same author (available via Amazon or Smashwords)

Motives, emotion and memory - exploring how doctors think
Proximity (Nina Charan medical thriller)
Extremis (2nd Nina Charan medical thriller)
The Pioneer
Malady/Therapy (short stories)

I would like to thank those Twitter followers who have recommended my blog to their own followers. Their positive feedback has kept me motivated, and the time that these busy people have taken to read my work has been both surprising and humbling. Special thanks to Kate Granger, Elin Roddy, Jonathon Tomlinson, Anne Cooper, Chris Rosevere and Katherine Sleeman.

INTRODUCTION 4

IN THE MACHINE 6

A NIGHT IN THE SYSTEM 7
5 DAYS: A TALE OF ESCALATION CREEP 14
INTERSECTION 19
AUTONOMY AND NECESSITY: 10 SCENES 22

SELF PRESERVATION 28

THE NEEDLE AND THE DAMAGE DONE 29
TOO CLOSE: FROM EMPATHY TO OVER-IDENTIFICATION 33
RAINSTORM 36

THE SILENT PATIENT 43

I HEAR YOU 44
DON'T TELL ME THE ODDS 48
SIGNS 52

THE APPRENTICESHIP 54

FADE TO GREEN 55
THE MOMENT: A TALE OF THREE DOCTORS 58
FATE NIGHT 66
THE EYES AND THE EARS: WHY ADAM BLEW THE WHISTLE 72
THE CUSP: ETHICS OF THE LEARNING CURVE 77
BLAMING PATIENTS: A VERY HUMAN TEMPTATION 84

NHS1 94

NHS2 ON THE YEAR 2053: A SIDEWAYS LOOK AT THE FUTURE 95
PRECIOUS: A LEGACY OF UNDERSTAFFING IN HEALTHCARE 104
JOURNEYMEN: WHY AREN'T DOCTORS MORE LOYAL TO THE NHS? 108

NEAR THE END 113

AN OPAQUE CODE: THE LIVERPOOL CARE PATHWAY AND A GAP IN PERCEPTION 114
A NEW WAY OF SAYING GOODBYE? (ON TWITTER) 119
SIGNALS: THE LANGUAGE OF UNCERTAINTY 120
SUBSTITUTES 125

Introduction

Since publishing the last collection of posts in *Motives, emotion and memory - exploring how doctors think* I have asked myself – where am I going with this? What is the common thread?

These posts came from a desire to explain how doctors arrive at medical decisions. They required a degree of honesty and a willingness to enter into uncomfortable areas of human motivation. For instance *The moment: a tale of three doctors* focuses on the place of reputation when considering how actively to advocate for a patient, and *The eyes and the ears: why Adam blew the whistle* (a sequel to *Why Michael didn't blow the whistle: pub scene*) exposes the personal concerns that must be balanced against the right course of action. In *Signals: the language of uncertainty* I look at language, at the way doctors try to communicate their fears for patients without actually saying so – a form of self-protection. Overt self-preservation from the emotional challenges that a career in medicine present, lies at the heart of *Too close: from empathy to over-identification* and *The needle and the damage done*. *Rainstorm* (the most popular so far as judged by 'page hits') imagines a demotivated junior doctor on the brink of resigning. Why? - the thickening atmosphere of direct accountability in the post-Francis Report, post-Mid Staffs era. He must learn how to function in a world where errors or omissions can no longer be ignored with a 'that's just how things are' attitude.

But an inquiring approach to the medical mindset does not explain the posts in which I tried to imagine what patients might be thinking, such as *Signs, Don't tell me the odds* or *I hear you*. These are complete fictions, as I have never been a genuinely ill patient at risk of death, and I have never been trapped in bed unable to communicate. But nor have most doctors (especially young ones), so the value of these exercises in imagination, or 'hyper-empathy' might be in demonstrating how *we* believe *they*, are responding to the day to day challenges of being on the ward. They are also valuable in demonstrating how far doctors can go in trying to understand what their patients are thinking as we interact with them; do they see through our prevarications or justifications for delays or errors?

Then there are the reflections on chance and hazard. *Intersection* looks at how patients who never see or know each other actually influence each other's fate. *Fate night* examines how a young doctor's social plans are scuppered by a series of unfortunate events, such that she must decide whether to stay or go, and *A night in the system* shows how a relative must assert herself to make the apparently oblivious, disconnected machine that is a hospital work for a patient.

And as in the last volume, I have written longer pieces on practical medical ethics that reference freely available resources on the internet, such as *The cusp: ethics of the learning curve*, *Blaming patients: a very human temptation* and *Substitutes* (which is about who we ask when trying to discover what incapacitous patients would have wanted.)

Finally there are several more political pieces, an arena in which I do not feel very comfortable as a doctor who spends more time looking down at the individual level than across at the societal level. Nevertheless, *Journeymen: why aren't doctors more loyal to the NHS*, *Precious: a legacy of understaffing* and *NHS2 in year 2053* are honest reactions to recent events.

So, returning from that quick tour, where am I actually going with this? The answer is…across a divide. That is my ambition. In *An opaque code: the Liverpool Care pathway and a gap in perception* I discuss a 'perception gap'. It is this gulf of understanding between doctors and their patients, and their patients' families, which drives many of the controversies that we see in medical practice. Poorly understood motives, failures in trust, insufficient accounting for the inevitable human frailties that lie behind some of our doctors' and nurses' actions or omissions. The articles in this book were written to shed light on those motivations and behaviours that directly affect patients. I hope they are good enough to serve as bricks in the fine bridge that others (such as Jonathon Tomlinson in his wonderful blog A Better NHS, or Kate Granger in her position as doctor, patient and generous communicator) began long before I started writing.

Phil Berry
December 2013

In the machine

A night in the system

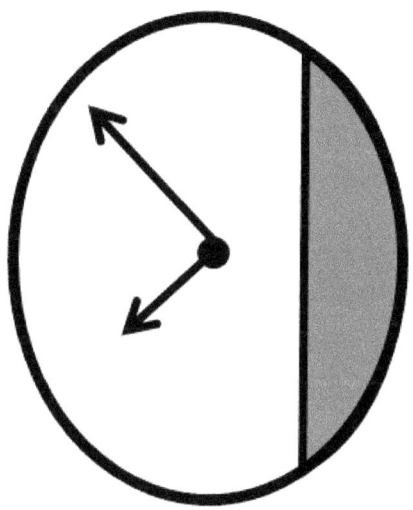

Introduction

This fictional scenario examines what patients, friends or relatives perceive when they enter the complex system that is a hospital. It describes what happens to a patient through the eyes of a friend who insists on staying with her overnight, and through the eyes of the junior doctor who is called to review her.

My intention is to portray processes and thoughts in a way that explains why things don't always look patient centred. For it is this expectation, of individualised care that is exquisitely responsive to any change in condition, that soon melts into a puddle of resigned disillusionment when ill patients struggle for attention in the apparent chaos of a busy ward. This scenario is about how the needs of the one must be balanced with the needs of the many, and how providing a safe environment for all might lead to less than 'ideal' care for the individual. It is also about how patients and relatives must find a balance between respectful passivity - blind faith in the system - or arm waving, vocal conspicuousness. While the patient and their family will be concerned about one very special person, the organisation must find a way of ordering, prioritising and allaying numerous disparate concerns. Thus the concept of 'acceptable' care versus 'ideal' care is invoked - or compromise.

Friend: I insisted that I stay with her. She was disorientated and upset, and I could not be sure that the staff on the ward would notice if she needed anything. At 9pm she rolled onto her side and fell asleep, at last. It had been a long and tiring day. Having made myself unpopular by breaking the rules on visiting hours I decided to keep to my head down, to be as invisible as possible. But I was glad I was there. I could hear her sniffles and moans, I could ask her what she wanted – whereas the nurses would come only if she pressed the buzzer (which had been placed near her hand, but which she didn't really understand). I watched and listened as other patients called out, and realised that it was necessary to call out repeatedly to attract attention. The nurses were moving incessantly, receiving new patients or administering drugs. This was an admissions ward, for fresh, potentially unstable patients. I understood that.

Doctor: I had seen her already, the patient and her friend. I had taken the initial history, performed the examination, arranged the admission. The friend was there in the ED, watchful, untrusting. She had that look – informed by a hundred scare stories in the media or a bad personal experience, I could tell she was convinced that hospitals were lethal, that there could be no guarantee of good care. I tried to reassure her; in fact I spent more time on her than I did on the patient, who was delirious. She asked if she could stay the night, and I said she would need to check with the ward sister.

Friend: When she began to moan I got worried. After about ten minutes I looked up and tried to find a nurse. The two main ones walked past quite a few times, by they were clearly busy, heads down, focussing on the problem in hand. I couldn't make eye contact – it reminded me of being in a restaurant. So I pressed the buzzer. The nurse came, and I was embarrassed by the orange light that flashed on the wall above the head of the bed. The nurse, he was a charge nurse, reached over to deactivate the light, slapping the button. He asked me what the matter was. I reported the groaning. He measured the blood pressure and pulse, tried to rouse her, but she wouldn't answer. Probably tired, he suggested. I had to agree...I couldn't exactly disagree, could I?

Doctor: I got bleeped about her a midnight. The nurse said her friend kept asking for her to be seen because she was making strange noises. But he couldn't tell me anything specific, there was nothing objectively abnormal to get worried about. But the nurse, Andy, said he wanted a medical review…and 'nurse concern' is a reason to go and check on patients. I agreed, and added her to my list.

Friend: I thought really hard about what to do next. I knew what I wanted – to drag the nurse over, or drag a doctor over. But I was nervous. Why? Because I was outside my comfort zone, I was surrounded by people more expert than myself, people who knew what to do. My role was supportive, not to act as some kind of alarm. And I was aware also that Mary was one of many, that her needs had to fit in with the needs of others. I didn't want to act selfishly. The system knew that something was wrong with Mary – and now the system, the hospital, would deal with it. What would I achieve by going on and on? Perhaps I would actually disadvantage her, by annoying the nurse, who would annoy the doctor by ringing again… I had done my bit. And then…my thoughts ran the other way. Who cared if I made myself unpopular, who cared if I challenged the system and annoyed the staff? – It wasn't about me, it was about Mary, and a threat to her health. Of course I didn't know at the time what was actually happening to her. If I had, I would have been screaming down the ward, demanding attention until they came.

Doctor: I was annoyed. Three bleeps for the same problem. OK, if there is new information it is justifiable to update me, but I cannot commit to reviewing patients, or reassuring their friends or families, just because they ask more frequently or insistently than the next patient. If that was the case then only the most vociferous would be seen, and others, with equally serious problems, would be disadvantaged. I have a feeling that the loudest do actually get the better care, and I'm sure many of my colleagues would agree with that. It's expedient, after all, to placate as soon as possible those who keep asking to see you. But I *do* get annoyed if I feel a family is dominating the ward or the nurses.

Friend: It was I who suggested to the charge nurse that Mary needed to see a doctor. Tiredness just doesn't do to a person what she was doing. Sighing, twitching, moaning. But still her observations seemed appropriate, her blood pressure and oxygen levels safe. I made up my own mind that whatever was wrong with her, it was beyond the ability of the nurse to make a diagnosis. I wasn't being offensive; it's just what I thought. I probably came across badly, but I had decided not to care about that.

Doctor: I actually checked her blood results again on the ward where I was spending most on the night; there were one of two that hadn't been ready when I saw her initially. I checked the kidney function, but it was normal. Blood glucose, normal. I mentally de-prioritised her. I had seen her x-ray already, and it was fine. I had taken a blood gas, and that too was fine. I couldn't think of any good reason why she should be getting sicker.

Friend: After ninety minutes of waiting for the doctor I became really agitated. The charge nurse looked over to me once or twice, then turned back to his monitor, or whatever he was working on. My thoughts were thus - He knows I'm worried, he's made the phone call to the doctor. It's up to the doctor now to decide how soon Mary should be seen. The situation hasn't changed, there's no point in me hassling them. The doctor – presumably the same one who saw us in Casualty – has lots to do. He knows about Mary. He knows how urgently, or not, she needs to be seen. I veered between frustration, caused by the lack of action, and calm, in the knowledge that the doctor was on his way.

Doctor: I heard nothing for a few hours. I should have gone down, I said I would, but I began to assume the situation had sorted itself out.

Friend: My anxiety grew. I was watching Mary minute by minute, and she wasn't right. I shook her a bit, poked her, tried to wake her. It looked like she wanted to be awake but couldn't talk. One eye opened. So I stood up again and approached the nearest nurse. It was a different one this time, the male nurse had gone off somewhere. Look, I said, I'm really worried. She in some sort of coma, or having a fit. 'The doctor is coming.' she said. That was two hours ago, I replied, could you call him again? She accompanied me back to the bed space. Can you try to wake her? I asked. She tried, but Mary wouldn't come round. I saw the fear rise in her, the sudden realisation that something was actually wrong. Perversely, I experienced a sudden rush of satisfaction, or vindication.

Doctor: The nurse, Jaya, bleeped me, and this time there was definitely something wrong. The patients conscious level was low, she couldn't talk. But it still didn't make sense. I promised to come down in the next half hour.

Friend: It was another 45 minutes; I timed it. When he came, after he had examined Mary, he adopted exactly the same expression – one of contained emergency, eyes wide and hyper-alert, while he worked out in his own mind what to do. He asked me if Mary had had a fall recently, and I said yes, a week ago. They hadn't asked before, it didn't seem like an important fact. She had only become ill over the last two days. The doctor began making phone calls…another doctor came, an anaesthetist in her scrubs, and they decided together that it was safe for Mary to go to the scanner.

Doctor: I didn't know about the fall. If I had, well, I'm not sure it would have made me examine her any earlier. There was no real evidence of worsening neurological status until the nurse on the ward calculated a formal coma score.

Friend: They told me that there was a blood clot on her the brain, and that it must have been accumulating slowly since the fall. Then they disappeared again, made more phone calls, and at 8 o'clock in the morning Mary was transferred to a neurosurgery unit. They drilled a hole in her skull, drained the blood, and sent her back three days later. She's still not right. She hasn't been herself since, no longer articulate, no longer interested in her Trollope, not the same.

Doctor: We recognised it pretty quickly, in my opinion. And they took her for decompression, which they don't always do. I've heard that she hasn't recovered that well. How did I hear? It was in the complaint. Her friend complained that there was undue delay in diagnosing the subdural.

Friend: I complained. I think – and I've asked several doctors of my acquaintance – that the hours that passed between my first alarm, my first comment to the charge nurse that she wasn't right, and the scan, contributed to her brain injury. I'm sure of it. And I ask myself, every single day, what if I had made more of a fuss, what if I had jumped up and down, dragged the nurse over, demanded that something be done four hours earlier? She would have had the scan, they would have found the clot, been transferred for the operation…all those brain cells could have been saved. I should have done more. I was there.

Doctor: I saw the letter, I was asked to comment on it for the Trust response.

Excerpt from response to complaint letter:

...after careful review by experts in the field, we have concluded that Mrs. Steven's diagnosis was made in a timely manner, and that surgery would not have been performed earlier even if the brain scan had been done on the evening of xx/xx/xx rather than the early hours of xx/xx/xx. Based on an independent review of the notes and observations during the night in question there appears to be no evidence of negligence by medical or nursing staff. A clinical decision to perform regular (e.g. hourly) neurological observations had not been made by the admitting doctor or the consultant who reviewed her the same evening, and the observations that were made (e.g. pulse, blood pressure) were done adequately...

Friend: So it seems there was no chance of her being treated earlier. Or no need. That's what it says. But I still disagree. If they had heard and understood my concerns, and if the penny had dropped about the fall and the bump on the head, I'm sure they would have done the scan and transferred her several hours earlier. But the system says that all was done correctly. I ask myself, what would have happened if I hadn't been there, if I hadn't badgered the nurse in the way I did? They would not have realised how ill she was until they tried to wake her up for breakfast. Hours later. Even more precious hours.

Doctor: Bottom line is, in my opinion, the patient's friend spent the night in the system, watching and worrying, rather than trusting. So every perceived delay became significant to her, and was translated into potential harm to the patient. When the gravity of Mary's condition became clear she saw how worried *I* was, how worried the *nurse* was, and interpreted that as an admission of our failure to make the diagnosis earlier. But there is always delay between the onset of a medical condition and its diagnosis, of course there is. Signs take time to develop, observations take time to become deranged. The question is, was the delay acceptable? Was it way outside reasonable expectation? I don't think it was in Mary's case. If...if...I had taken a better history and had known that she had fallen and hit her head a week before, I might have put her on neuro obs [hourly checks, as mentioned in the letter], but as she didn't appear 'neurological' when I saw her, I might not have. Overnight we don't expect nurses to check a patient's conscious level thoroughly every time they do blood pressures, because patients sleep. I am pretty sure that if Mary's friend hadn't been there we would have made the diagnosis in the same time frame. She didn't need to be there. What her presence did was highlight, to her, how busy we all are, and how we cannot hope to attend to each patient frequently and immediately. No system can offer that.

Friend: I visited her yesterday. She's in a nursing home now. I still regret what I didn't do. If I had followed my instincts, made a hell of a fuss, the old Mary would still be there to chat with me. I'm sure of it.

5 days: a tale of escalation creep

Day 1 A 90 year old lady, Mrs V, is admitted to hospital with symptoms of pneumonia. She was managing at home 6 months ago but has become increasingly dependent on her family; the plan was to employ or arrange carers soon. She always said she never wanted strangers around – the words 'fiercely independent' are used a lot. She saw her husband die on an intensive care five years ago – it was very unpleasant, and her son makes it clear from the outset that she would never want to be put on a ventilator. Treatment begins, and her son actively engages the consultant in a DNAR conversation during the post-take ward round. All are agreed she should not be subjected to it should her heart stop. But the consultant explains that the pneumonia is not that severe, and says she is optimistic that Mrs V will improve. The son was due to go on a business trip for three days – he asks if that is wise. The consultant says,

"Well, nothing is ever certain, but her oxygen levels are not too bad, and she has no other illnesses. I can't tell you what you should do, but she doesn't seem to be in imminent danger."

He leaves.

Day 2: Mrs V appears confused to the registrar who does the daily ward round. He notes that her oxygen level is borderline. The oxygen flow is turned up, the level improves. But later that day it dips again (saturation 83% on an oxygen mask). The registrar calls the consultant,

"I was thinking about some non-invasive ventilation on the medical HDU."

"That would be reasonable. Her son was keen not to medicalise too much…"

"I think she just needs a couple of days of support."

"I agree. She was pretty good before, the antibiotics haven't really kicked in yet. Any positive microbiology?"

"Streptococcal antigen positive."

"Ah. Well at least we know. But it could be aggressive. I'm happy for you to arrange transfer."

Day 3: Mrs V has spent the night on a tight fitting mask which allows oxygen to enter the lungs under pressure. She struggles with the mask periodically, but settles eventually. Her oxygen levels are better, but she is still confused. The team put this down to delirium, an acute confusional state. A blood sample is drawn from the wrist, and it shows that her carbon dioxide levels have risen. The HDU nurse asks if the team could arrange an arterial line, a cannula inserted into the radial (wrist) artery, to allow more frequent blood sampling. This will avoid repeated needles. The registrar agrees, the SHO volunteers. He can feel the artery easily, and is confident. The ward round moves on and the SHO stays behind, but 40 minutes later he calls the registrar.

"I couldn't get it in."

"How many attempts?"

"Just three…but it bled and she has a big bruise."

"Leave it for now. I'll do it."

Day 4: The consultant does a ward round in the morning.

"How come she's got a nasogastric tube?" she asks of the charge nurse.

"She was sick overnight. Her stomach filled with gas because of the positive pressure. She's a lot more comfortable now."

"Is she eating?"

"Not much. She has some sips during breaks off the mask."

The team look at the arterial blood sample results. Gradually, with the eye of faith, the respiratory failure is improving. Mrs V cries out. She has pleurisy, intense pain at the edge of the lungs. Simple pain killers are not enough, and she is prescribed morphine. As the consultant walks away she notices the urinary catheter bag hanging from a stand.

"Why the catheter?" she asks. The charge nurse replies,

"She couldn't manage with the commode, not on the mask. She's high risk for pressure sores. We put it in yesterday."

Day 5: Mrs V deteriorates. A repeat x-ray shows that the pneumonia has spread further through the right lung. The registrar calls the consultant.

"I've got quite a bad feeling about her now. I think her age is beginning to tell, I know she didn't have any other illnesses but…"

"You're right. Once things begin to go downhill it's hard to see her getting better."

"I understand her son didn't want her to go to intensive care."

"I don't think they would take her to be honest. But yes, he told me that she wouldn't want that. In fact he needs to know what's going on. He's supposed to be coming back today."

"The nurse called him this morning. He arrived back in the country in the early hours apparently. He's on his way in."

"I'll speak to him. We need to discuss de-escalation."

At 2pm her son arrives on the ward. He finds his mother lying on her bed, barely conscious now. She is muttering words but he cannot understand them. A monitor pings and alarms insistently above her head. Trailing from her body are a urinary catheter, an arterial line transducer, two intravenous infusion lines and the wide oxygen tube attached to the mask at her face. The air and oxygen in the mask whistles. Cardiac monitoring leads trail out of her gown into the machine that is alarming. He sees the bruise on her forearm that has now developed into a 4-inch haematoma that sits proud to the skin. He pushes the curtain aside, tears in his eyes, storms out of the cubicle and shouts in the direction of the nurses' station,

"WHO DID THIS? SHE NEVER WANTED THIS!"

She dies later in the day, the mask having been removed and the monitor having been turned off. Six weeks later her son writes to complain about the inappropriate, overly intensive treatment to which she was subjected during her final illness.

What happened here?

*

I wrote this to explain how, as the cliché goes, the 'road to hell is paved with good intentions'. Looking back, Mrs V's treatment seems misguided. How could her consultant have allowed a frail 90 year old lady with (what proved to be) severe pneumonia undergo multiple, potentially painful and distressing procedures to no avail? Didn't she hear the son when he explained how Mrs V had witnessed her husband undergo a similar ordeal? Why didn't she put a brake on the system and stop the medical rollercoaster in its tracks?

But then, let's go back to beginning and follow these events step by step. The infection didn't look that bad at the beginning, there was little reason to expect Mrs V's death. So, when Mrs V's oxygen levels fell, a judgment was made that a short period of assisted ventilation would help. But then, to avoid repeated blood tests, an arterial line was required – a procedure that proved harder than it looked. The gastric tube had to be passed, the nurses couldn't just stand by as her stomach filled with gas. The catheter was routine. Every step was justified.

How could this have been avoided? Well, if the son had been there every day he may have called a halt to things, but I'm not sure he would have felt able to question each procedure in the face of enthusiasm and almost routine pattern following on the part of junior doctors and nurses. So to stop this we need to go back further…to the initial conversation. It needed to focus on the 'ceiling of care'.

Perhaps the consultant should have made a decision, in discussion with the son, that whatever happened Mrs V would remain on the basic medical ward…even if she deteriorated. In that way there would be no danger of being prescribed the mask, and no danger of having to endure the paraphernalia that can goes with it. The son would have returned (perhaps a day or too earlier if he had been contacted about the deterioration) to find his mother being treated on the original ward, in relative comfort. Knowing how things turned out in the end, that decision would have been right. But no-one knew how things were going to go. The consultant thought there was a chance of survival. She decided that the burden of treatment was reasonable in this case, despite the caution that the patient's son had expressed. She made the wrong call.

I have no right answer here. I wish only to highlight that, as Soren Kierkegaard said, *'Life can only be understood backwards; but it must be lived forwards.'*

Intersection

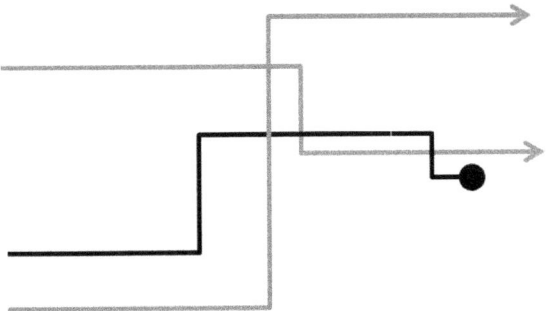

This is a brief tale of two patients who never met, but whose lives became briefly entwined with huge consequences. Until the day that saw both became ill their life lines had not intersected before. Suddenly those lines veered from their usual course and dived across the city towards a bland, anonymous nexus...the hospital. They arrived within an hour of each other but were too preoccupied with their own symptoms and fears to become aware of one another in adjacent cubicles. Their relatives passed in the corridor, and may have stood in line together at the coffee machine. The patients, an elderly man and a thirty-five year old woman, were seen by different doctors. His angina settled with morphine, oxygen and nitrates; her asthma attack eased with nebulisers and infusions. She was transferred to the medical high dependency ward for monitoring, he to the coronary care unit. Their lives diverged once again as they were transported to different ends of the hospital.

At 2am his angina leapt back up for attention. The nurse looking after him turned up the nitrate infusion, but bleeped the doctor on call as the pain score rose from 7 to 9. The doctor responded and began to make his way to the ward. He knew that the ECG was essentially unchanged - the nurse had told him so, and he trusted her interpretation. She had seen a hundred times more ischaemic ECGs in her career than he had. But he had a plan - intravenous beta blockers, to slow the heart and make the myocardium less hungry for oxygen.

As he turned the penultimate corner his bleep went off again. He spotted a phone hanging from the wall and called the number. It was HDU. A young woman with new onset asthma was deteriorating. Oxygen saturations were dropping, she was confused, peak flows were unrecordable...every red flag he could think of was being waved.

The coronary care nurse knew what needed to be done. Her patient's pulse was 95 beats per minute, but a simple injection could bring it down to 65 and ease the pain. He was clutching his chest, pressing on the sternum as though to reach into the cavity and tear the source from his body. And now, on the cardiac monitor, she saw definite signs of ischaemia. Where was that doctor?

The doctor turned the final corner...and entered the high dependency unit. The asthma patient was close to collapse. He laid her down, began to assist her breathing with a bag and mask, and calmly ordered the nearest nurse to summon the entire medical emergency team.

On the cardiac ward the nurse had gone so far as to draw up the beta blocker in readiness. She was quite prepared to tell the doctor what to do if necessary. Then she would phone the on-call cardiologist herself to discuss emergency angioplasty. Nervous now, she walked from the bed space to the desk, in order to bleep him again. He had said he was on his way, and, though she couldn't be sure, she thought she had heard his footsteps approach up the corridor five minutes ago. He must have got distracted.

'Good call,' said the anaesthetist on the emergency team, '...she needed intubating. I'm glad you didn't hang about.' The junior doctor felt good for what he done. He had recognised the red flags and had responded to them efficiently. As he left this scene of minor glory (he had qualified only 18 months ago after all) the crash bleep sounded. He and the rest of the crash team ran to coronary care, leaving behind only the anaesthetist who continued to ventilate the asthma patient.

They worked on the elderly angina patient for 25 minutes, but his heart could not be coaxed back into life. The many injuries it had accumulated before and since the bypass operation 18 years ago meant, for reasons we don't fully understand, that once its lifelong habit of beating had been interrupted it would not be restarted.

His family were shocked, but not surprised, if that combination of reactions makes sense. They knew nothing of the junior doctor's genuine intention to see their father, nor of the badly timed phone call that caused him to turn around and walk away from the coronary care unit. There is no way of knowing if his arrival would have made a difference...but it might have. So here we see how the life lines of two patients eventually crossed, the exact point of intersection being in that corridor, where the beige plastic phone hung on the wall, when the doctor on call decided to prioritise the needs of one before the needs of another.

A hospital represents a huge exchange in which hundreds and thousands of life lines touch each other every minute, altering in subtle ways the medical decisions, therapeutic actions and clinical outcomes of complete strangers. This sounds strange...and not a little wrong. A patient's outcome should depend on several things, but not on the nature of their neighbour's competing condition! On any given day the care a patient receives will be influenced not only by the vagaries of their own illness, the expertise of the doctor they encounter and the compassion of the staff they meet, but by numerous factors beyond the essential medical dynamic. The concentration and character of life lines running through the great nexus will also determine what happens. This fanciful representation may reveal a degree of caprice that we would rather not admit to, but we witness caprice every day, in nature and disease, in human response, in physiological or pharmacological idiosyncrasy. It is unavoidable. While we marshal these random factors into a logical, safe and personal management plan to the best of our ability, it does no harm to remind ourselves that the job of picking apart those life lines and prioritising their needs can never be an exact science.

Autonomy and necessity: 10 scenes

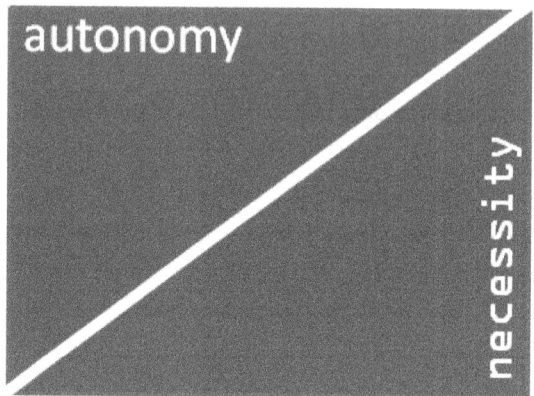

Scene 1 - Café

Am I happy with the care I received? Nothing turned out as I had foreseen, little was done to me that I actually wanted. Choices…don't make me laugh. The only choice that would have made any difference would have been the choice not to have this illness. And who has that choice?

Scene 2 – Clinic (a year earlier)

Will it go away?

It's a chronic condition…long term. It can get better, or go into remission, sometimes for a very long time, but there will always be the risk that it will come back. And sometimes it can get a lot worse…

In what way?

If the bowel becomes dangerously inflamed it can make you very ill, and the types of medication required to calm it down are correspondingly very strong.

But it doesn't have to be removed?

Sometimes. Sometimes it does.

What?

Colectomy, removal of the bowel, is sometimes needed. But the way you have been up 'til now, it doesn't seem likely that you will be one of those patients. I'm confident we can use medication to keep things under control.

You have to. I cannot have a bag. I cannot.

Scene 3 – Emergency Department

How long have you had colitis?

Three months now. It was all going so well.

Who are you under?

Dr Jackson.

And is he thinking about changing your treatment?

He did, three weeks ago. What are you going to recommend now?

You need a few days in hospital, we need to get the inflammation under control again.

Scene 4 – Ward

Well Susan, the injections have worked! It's time to get home.

It was close, wasn't it?

Yes. Another two days and we would have had to recommend surgery.

Scene 5 – Clinic

I'm not right Dr Jackson. I'm never normal any more. I'm losing my hair on this drug…

It's unusual to lose...

Well I am, OK! And I've taken weeks and weeks off work this year…

Susan, you know what we need to talk about don't you. Let me refer you to one of my surgical colleagues, Miss Baker, she's very good, very understanding…

No. I don't want it! Anything but that.

I have to discuss your case in one of our meetings anyway. We all meet up and look at the x-rays, the blood results. I can't see you going on like this indefinitely. And there are options, believe me.

I don't want you taking any decisions without me.

Don't worry, we won't.

Scene 6 - Meeting

There's only one outcome here Paul. She needs to accept that she has to lose her bowel. I'll have a chat with her. It's not uncommon…I'd try to put it off for as long as possible if it was me too.

OK, I'll ring her and tell her the offer is there. It's up to her.

Better to do it now than in an emergency. I could do it in one stage, laparoscopically. No bag.

Scene 7 – Clinic

So you see Susan, that's my advice. And that's the advice of the whole team.

I don't have a choice.

I wouldn't look at it like that. Your choices have shifted, to a different level. You no longer have the choice not to have surgery, but the type of surgery you have, and when, is still within your power. I know it doesn't sound like much, but that's all we can do…guide you through the options and ensure that you are as fully informed as possible. But we can't take the disease away.

Scene 8 -Ward (two weeks later)

So has it gone?

Has what gone Susan?

The one stage option? Avoiding the bag?

I'm afraid so. The bowel has deteriorated, we can't make the pouch safely without giving you some time to improve, with a stoma. I'm sorry.

It's exactly what I wanted to avoid. My husband… (Susan weeps)

This time next year Susan, it will be over. All healed. Not normal, I accept that, but you'll feel so much better.

But why can't Miss Baker do it? I know her, I trust her…

We can't wait for her to come back from holiday. It's not exactly an emergency now, but it's getting that way. The operation has to be done before the weekend. You've been on these infusions for a week now, they begin to affect the way the body heals. And for the last two days there has been no sign of improvement in the inflammation. It's time to remove that colon.

I don't *want* an operation.

Susan, you have to consent to it. For it to go ahead you must sign the consent form. Is your husband coming in this afternoon?

Yes.

I'll come back to the ward then.

To gang up on me you mean…

Scene 9 – Ward, next day

So these are the options Susan. I'm sure Miss Baker ran through some of them with you when you spoke to her in the clinic. I can't predict what I'll find when I start the operation, but if it's not too damaged I can either do this (points to one of the pictures he has drawn), or this…

(Susan looks away) I don't *care* anymore. Just do what you have to do. I feel so ill, I can't decide. It's up to you.

Scene 10 – Café (present day)

And that's how it was. All those choices, those shared decisions, in the end I just said – *get on with it! You know best!* My disease didn't respect choices, it accelerated, deteriorated, pushed me around, took away my autonomy. *Me!* Someone who had always, always insisted that she was in control! The irony of it.

And you've coped, with the stoma bag?

I cope with everything life throws at me. Of course. Next week I go in for the reversal. And in some ways I am less demanding now… I know they'll look after me, they'll do what they have to do. I can't choose how Miss Baker does the operation, how she stitches…I can't choose what kind of ward I go into, who I am next to, if the nurses and juniors are nice to me. The choices they talk about are, in my experience, not choices at all. They are theoretical. They are forks in the road that look equivalent from a distance, but when you get there, if you are travelling at speed, you have little or no say about which one you go down. To resist the momentum, in whichever direction it seems to be taking you - and by momentum I mean the opinion of your doctor, of the team - is foolish. It's unsafe. Better to give in to it, believe what they say, trust them. But that's just my experience. Don't take my word for it.

Self preservation

The needle and the damage done

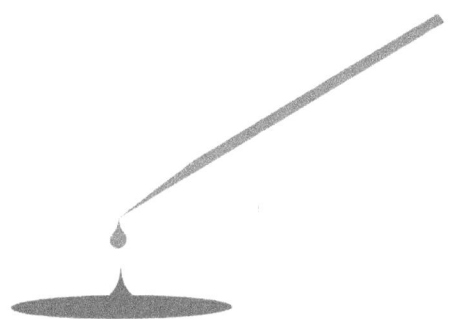

Scrolling through my timeline on Twitter the other day, I saw that a junior doctor had suffered a 'blood splash', presumably in the face. This is when a patient's blood is sprayed or flicked into your mouth or eyes...carrying with it the risk of infection from a blood borne virus such as hepatitis C or HIV (medical staff are immunised to hepatitis B). It made me think back on a similar experience as a junior doctor...a needle stick injury from a patient infected with hepatitis C. I'll describe what happened in a minute, not because I enjoy telling unpleasant personal stories, but because I think the impact that these 'avoidable but let's face it they're going to happen now again' accidents have on doctors and nurses should be understood and emphasised. When I looked into the subject I discovered that research had been published on the subject this year, the results of which I will go on to summarise. It seems that the psychological impact of these accidents can be very grave indeed.

*

As soon as I felt the deep sting of the needle as it entered my finger I knew what it meant - potential disaster. I was cutting a space between the ribs of a patient on intensive care, making room for the insertion of a large chest drain. The tissues were tough, and I had to tear at the fibres with my fingers deep under the skin. But the patient was not sedated, and she was feeling it despite the local anaesthetic injection I had administered beforehand. So I did something stupid. I kept one finger in the cut, so as not to lose the track I had struggled to form, and with my other hand I carefully inserted the anaesthetic needle alongside it. In this way I hoped to numb the deeper tissues. I jabbed my own fingertip – *ouch*...a shock, but not really painful. It was the knowledge that hepatitis C viruses in my patient's blood could now be running up the veins of my arm and into my bloodstream that caused me to freeze in fear. I withdrew my finger, looked down at my hand, tore off the glove, and squeezed the fingertip until droplets came out. The nurse who had been helping me recognised what had happened, but had nothing to say. I walked over to a sink, washed the blood off, wrapped a waterproof dressing around the tiny wound and went back to the patient. She still needed a chest drain after all. Soon the job was done, and the rest of the nightshift passed without incident. But throughout the small hours I could think only of myself: were there any viruses in the needle? How many would it take to cause a permanent infection? Would I need anti-viral treatment, would it work, could I continue to be a doctor while receiving the famously toxic combination of interferon and ribavirin? Might it fail, would I develop cirrhosis, would I end up in this very hospital, waiting for a transplant? Oh God.

I was distracted by anxiety for weeks, not to a disabling degree...not so as anyone would notice. At six weeks I had a blood test to see if there were detectable levels of virus in me. A week later I attended the occupational health department to get the result. The nurse had not read a Hep C result before, it seemed to me. She looked quizzically at the small piece of paper in front of her, and tilted her head slightly.

'Err...you have...err...Hepatitis C.'

I nearly fainted. I looked at the report closely, upside-down, and lunged forward,

'Let me see that!'

I turned the report round and saw that she had misread a < for a >. I had < 50 virus particles per millilitre of blood, not > 50! I was *negative*! She accepted my interpretation, and was embarrassed. I left the room and walked back to my ward. My skin was cold and wet. I felt fifteen years older.

There were antibody tests at three and six months, and they were negative too. I was not infected. In fact, looking back, knowing more now about the absolute risks, and the cleaning action that plastic gloves perform as a needle passes through them, it was never very likely. But the experience changed me.

*

Professor Ben Green and Emily Griffiths (University of Chester) recently published a paper called 'Psychiatric consequences of needle stick injury' in *Occupational Medicine*. They administered a depression questionnaire to 17 needle stick injury (NSI) recipients who had been badly affected enough to be referred to a psychiatric clinic. None were actually infected. They compared these results with 125 non-NSI recipients who had been referred for other forms of psychological trauma. The authors hypothesised that NSI caused shorter or less intense periods of psychological morbidity. Their findings included a description that I recognised immediately,

'Four of the cases (24%) described an initial period of up to 2 days of acute anxiety, disbelief, tremor and profound sleeplessness consistent with an acute stress reaction.'

Within the (admittedly highly selected) group of 17,

'Thirteen (76%)...had a diagnosis of adjustment disorder (AD). Four (24%) met the guidelines for post traumatic stress disorder according to ICD-10 diagnoses.'

Other observations included,

'NSI patients with AD repeatedly said that although accident and emergency staff or occupational health staff had reassured them that the chances of seroconversion were small they focused on the fact that there was still a 'possibility' of seroconversion and thus did not feel reassured.

They concluded, among other things, that

'psychiatric disorders in NSI patients were similar to other trauma-related psychiatric illness in severity, but while they last for 9 months on average, this was not as long as other psychiatric trauma patients. Psychiatric illness following NSIs had major impacts on work attendance, family relationships and sexual health.'

*

These individuals were at the worse end of the spectrum, and the conclusions reached in this paper do not apply to all NSI recipients. I wonder if there is a more subtle effect on those who do not end up being seen by a psychiatrist - a heightened, and more general, sense of self-preservation. My own experience brought it home to me that while my career would involve seeing hundreds or thousands of patients who might carry serious or incurable infections, there was only *one* of me. I resolved to do everything I could to protect myself...not to a paranoid degree, but by applying a greater sense of caution. So, instead of plunging into the next cardiac arrest situation without a care for the bodily fluids that were leaking onto the patient's chest or bed, I held back until my gloves were safely on. I know that's what you're supposed to do anyway, but in real life people don't. They rush to save the patient. When I saw a woman collapse during a night out in Soho I ran up to her, checked for a pulse, but did not contemplate performing mouth-to-mouth resuscitation without a mask. I felt selfish, but I could not face the prospect of waiting for more blood test results. (Mouth to mouth is out of fashion now anyway – and fortunately, she was breathing.) Beyond the arena of infection, I became less inclined to make sacrifices that might affect my health or put me at risk of making mistakes; swapping into crazy sequences of night and day shifts as a favour for colleagues, covering extra clinics when dog-tired...sensible behaviour, in no way abnormal, but a change. The damage done.

The Needle and the Damage Done is a song by Neil Young (Harvest, 1972)

Too close: from empathy to over-identification

I know what to do. Make sure I know exactly what the diagnosis is, speak confidently about the possible treatments, have an onward plan prepared to allow some positive focus, a constructive approach. He's bound to ask about prognosis but I'll have to deflect that…it's too early to get into numbers. He's going to need to see an oncologist. This is just the first hurdle – breaking the bad news. He has an inkling, I know, but we haven't talked about it openly. I know how to do this.

There will be a quiet, private room. There will be two seats, for him and his wife. I'm going to switch off my phone. The diary is clear for an hour, we can talk for as long as necessary. I've done it before, I've seen worse. It's not exactly routine but it's part of the job.

He's not much older than me. He shouldn't have something this serious. I think he's got young children. Last time I saw him he was on his own, on the ward. We drew some fluid and sent it off for analysis. This is a follow up appointment, arranged urgently after the report landed on my desk. I did mention some possibilities at the time, as I was suspicious even at that early stage. I've no idea if he shared his fears with his wife or partner. She's coming with him though.

What does he need from me? He's a fairly matter of fact man, he just wants to get to the facts. And that's how I'm going to be. I've got the facts, but I haven't got the whole story. I can't tell him how long he's got. But I can provide a clear interpretation of the facts that I do have. I've done it many times.

That I'm thinking so much about this means something. I tell people every week that they have potentially lethal diseases, but this one is bugging me. I think it's because he and I are similar. We're at similar stages in our different careers, we both have young families. Am I nervous because I fear for myself when I see him? Am I worried that his misfortune will contaminate me? What is going on if *my* response to *his* illness is concern for *my* own future? If bad luck was contagious I'd be dead by now.

It's different with the elderly; serious illness is an almost inevitable part of aging. And they tend to take it with little expressed emotion. What was it I read the other day? *'He had reached an age where death no longer has the quality of ghastly surprise...'* The Great Gatsby. A book about young people. This man is being halted in his prime. I find myself thinking about how I would react if it was me. I'm thinking about it too much, that's the problem.

I am walking to the clinic. It's pretty quiet in the department as I arranged to use a room over the lunch hour. They haven't arrived yet. I go through the notes, but there is no new information. A nurse opens the door and tells me he has arrived. He enters with his partner, they take their seats.

How are you? It's an irrelevant question, a needless pleasantry.

Okay. Have you got the results?

Yes. There are abnormal cells in the fluid. Cancer cells. His partner juts forward. You mean it's cancer?

Yes.

I look at him. He is sweating. He is no longer receptive to my words.

His phone vibrates. In a matter of fact way, as is his manner, he pulls it out of his jacket pocket to read the text. I think he's consciously carrying on as normal. I glance at the lighted screen of his phone, and see the image that he has saved to his home screen. Two children. I am rocked by the sudden realisation that he is not going to see them grow up. I stutter. I am very uncomfortable. The professionalism, the experience, the constructive momentum that I hoped would facilitate this consultation, have faded to nothing. I lose my way repeatedly, failing to find a secure path between his need for information and her evolving horror.

10 minutes later they leave. I have laid out the short-term plan, forced it onto the table, and I have avoided the big question about prognosis. But it didn't go well. I know it didn't go well. How could it, really? But my 'performance' was not right. For a few moments I was swimming in the murky waters of that couple's emotional pain, and I was not doing my job. Perhaps they noticed. She did, I'm pretty sure.

Empathy is vital in the practise of medicine. It involves understanding a patient's condition from their perspective. But it lies on a spectrum, with 'detached concern' at one end, and over-identification at the other. In this instance I over-identified. Next time I will play it cool. Think less. Feel less. Stay professional.

(This fictional episode was inspired by several clinical encounters.)

Rainstorm

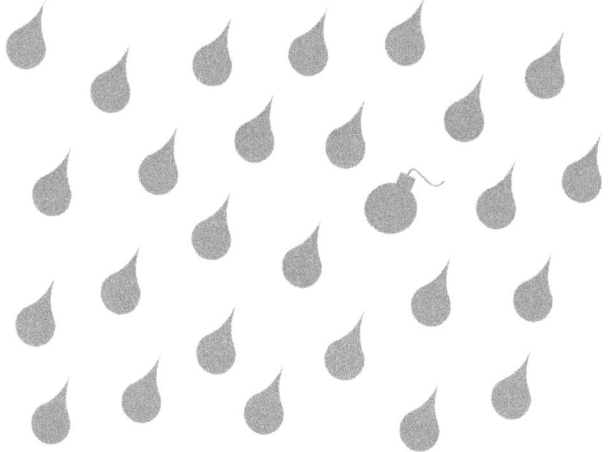

He had sat through the starter and the main course, each morsel sticking in his dry gullet. Opportunities had come and gone, but he had failed to take them, paralysed by cowardice. Nevertheless, his mind was made up and nothing was going to change his course. His mother seemed to sense that something was wrong; the conversation faltered, he declined to have his wine glass refilled.

"What's wrong love?"

"I'm giving up medicine."

oOo

A month earlier.

He parked his car and turned off the radio. --- '...*doctors will be criminalised if found guilty of wilful negligence...*' --- was the sentence echoing in his mind as he entered the hospital through a side door. He was on-call today, but he hoped to see some of his own patients before things began to heat up. His first patient had been diagnosed with inoperable lung cancer, and their relatives were on the ward waiting to talk to him. David took them into a private room. As he closed the door behind them the patient's daughter pre-empted him, asking,

"Who are you?"

"I'm David Clark, the SHO."

She opened a spiral bound note book and began to take notes.

"…before you go on doctor, can you tell me when you found the lump?"

"Well…soon after he came in, when he had the scan…"

"Wasn't it on the x-ray he had on the day he came to casualty?"

"Well yes, but we, the doctors looking after him them, were concentrating on the infection, but now a scan proved it…"

"That was two weeks ago. I don't understand why there has been a delay."

David controlled himself. His plan, the careful steps he rehearsed in order to take the family along an explanatory path of diagnosis, treatment options, arrangements, support…had been blown to bits. Flustered, he continued. Everything was being written down. A phrase from the cop shows rattled in his head as tried to focus on the words, *'…will be used against you in a court of law…'*

The day got busier. While he was inserting a urinary catheter he was fast bleeped to another ward. He couldn't move, committed to the task that he had begun. He hurried it, didn't do it quite as carefully as he normally would, anxious to leave the patient and rush to the emergency. When he got to the other ward a charge nurse informed him that he had no choice but to fill an incident form. Only the most junior member of the team had responded to the urgent call, and she hadn't been able to deal with the emergency.

"But I was tied up, I couldn't come…'

"I know doctor. But we have to do these forms. Otherwise nothing changes, does it…?'

He imagined his name in the text, the focus of culpability. In the Acute Medical Unit ward he received a call; the bed manager had been trying to find him. There was a patient on an outlying ward under his team's care who had not been reviewed for four days. Although

David was mired in emergency admissions by now (enjoying the rapid throughput of fresh cases, stimulated by the need to make fast decisions, arrange investigations and take responsibility for the treatment plans), he dragged himself away to visit the lost patient. She was very elderly, evidently succumbing to pneumonia on a background of heart disease. In fact the admitting team had done a very thorough job. They had spoken to the family, discussed resuscitation, introduced the idea of palliative care, but then…nothing. For four days. No doctors. The odd on-call visit to prescribe fluids, but nothing substantive. It shouldn't happen, but it can and it does. And now her son was here, visibly upset. David introduced himself. The son retorted,

"I want an explanation!"

"I'm sorry, there must have been a mix up, and then over the weekend…"

"I don't care. No-one has seen her, she's been ignored. Who is this?" He pointed to the consultant's name written in blue marker on the white sign above the bed, "Is he the consultant?"

"She. Yes she is. But your mother has only just come under her care."

"No she hasn't, that name has been up there every day. But you didn't see her on Monday or Tuesday. It's neglect. What chance she did have has been lost."

"The nurses tell me she has been comfortable."

"Yes, she has. But…

David entered the final hours of his difficult day. He made many accurate diagnoses and many good decisions. The consultant seemed happy with his clerking but David was down. He kept thinking back to the old lady's son, his sharp words. 'Wilful…' 'Ignored…' 'Neglected…' David's usual spark had been extinguished. His shift was over. As he walked into the doctors' room to pick up his coat the bleep went off one last time. He called the number.

"Dr Clark. Hi, it's Mary on Chestnut ward. Mr Threlfall, the man we put out a fast bleep for earlier, he's died. No, it was expected, your registrar came to see him and made him not for resuscitation. It's just, because of that incident form earlier, I'm going to send the notes on to the morbidity and mortality meeting for review. As a formality, you know.'

As he closed the door of the office behind him a colleague ran past him in the corridor; breathlessly he shouted,

"Crash call. Some guy who had a catheter inserted this morning, on Warfarin, he's bleeding out…"

David opened his car door, sat heavily in the seat, and turned on the radio. ---*'Police have confirmed a second criminal investigation into a potentially avoidable death in Mid Staffordshire, five years after…'*--- He turned it off, put his palms on the steering wheel and his forehead on the backs of his hands, and muttered, "I can't do this anymore."

oOo

David sat in his consultant's office. She had locked the door and asked that they not be disturbed. She had heard about his decision, and started by asking him to hear her out. Then she explored what it was that had made up his mind. He described his shift from hell. She said,

"I'll tell you what I think. We've got to help you adapt to these…stresses. The scrutiny, the incident reporting…"

"You mean just ignore it?"

"In a way, yes. They should not dictate how you function as a doctor. Because they are more visible – after Mid Staffs, after the Francis Report – and because they have imposed themselves on you, you have come to react to them rather than the instincts that drew you into this vocation in the first place. They are important, yes, they are there to protect patients, yes, but from those doctors who might be harmful. You are not one of those doctors. You are good. You should be able to function without bring fearful of running into these electric fences and getting hurt all the time. From what I've seen of the way you practice medicine, you will find a path goes nowhere near the edges of reasonable, sensible practice."

"Yet I seem to have run into those fences time and again. I described it to my girlfriend as living in a continuous rainstorm, where each raindrop is a new patient and a potential clinical incident or mistake that I must protect myself from. Usually I can, using my knowledge and experience, or luck, but sometimes one of those raindrop gets through, and explodes. And I never know which one it's going to be…"

"What happens to patients isn't always down to you or your decisions. Some get sick despite everything. You can't necessarily stop that, so you can't take the blame. Looking back, did you actually do anything wrong during that day on call?"

"I felt like I did. Incident forms, threats of 'wilful negligence'! And the catheter. That was my fault."

"Didn't you hear? He had a bladder tumour, that's why he bled! Forget that. And 'wilful negligence'…please don't be scared by that term. The relative who used it wasn't criticising you, he didn't know who you were. He was frustrated with the situation. Wouldn't you be? That term, whatever it means, wasn't designed to be applied to isolated mistakes."

"But she *was* neglected."

"Yes, by our system. And we've tried to close that gap. But not by you. You were never in danger. Did you really think you could go to jail? Really?"

"No. Yes. I don't know. I just kept hearing it…"

"I know. And the incident form…well, they are important, and are used to alert us – the doctors who will be working here for years! – about what needs to be fixed. That wasn't personal either."

"I appreciate what you're saying, I really do. But I can't work in this atmosphere of…negativity."

"But it's just that. An atmosphere. We have to learn to breathe it without taking it personally, without a sense of suffocation.."

"So it's my fault – this crisis. I've got it out of perspective?"

"A bit. That's why we're talking. I want to help you understand how a good doctor must accept that they will be subject to what seems like criticism now and again. You seem to be aware of your limitations. In fact you may be too aware, because you've grown nervous of them. The warnings and safety nets that have become so much more visible recently are not there to punish you. If you, as one of the great majority of trainee doctors who are good, intelligent and conscientious, are picked out and quoted in some incident form, or referred to anonymously in a mortality meeting, it's more likely to be a reflection of how stressed the service is, or how fallible a particular system is. It's not a judgment on you."

"But if I am a good doctor why am I being reminded about these systems all the time? Threatened by them."

"There is a temptation to use them as levers, to get you to see patients more urgently than you, as the doctor, might feel is appropriate. Remember, you are the doctor, your opinion is valuable .If you are asked to see someone who is deteriorating, you have the right, by virtue of your experience and understanding of clinical priorities, to decide how soon they should be seen. But if somebody else thinks they should be seen sooner, and they are able to wield a stick, it's natural for them to do this to motivate you to hurry up. They want their patient seen first – that's natural. But in doing so they ensure that you are driven by a negative motivation rather a positive one. You fear the situation rather than embrace it. And look where it has brought you."

"So I just say no, sorry, I'll come when I want to."

"If you are juggling what appear to be equally important priorities, yes. But you must explain why, help the person you are talking to understand and, if possible, agree. And you must follow through, see that patient, hold your course, finish each task that you begin, and leave the ward confident that you have dealt with the problem in hand…"

"And when I get called away to see an even sicker patient…"

"Ask, build a picture, make your own mind up. Things don't happen that fast. The sicker patient will have been deteriorating all night, they can usually wait another ten minutes. If they are arresting you will find out, there will be a crash call. It's all about accommodating the continuous stream of emergencies, catching the raindrops, without being caught up and carried away in the flow. If you do you will become disorientated. You are the one who needs to keep calm, maintain perspective. It's you they're looking to for reassurance. Remember that David."

"I hadn't thought about it like that. I've just felt…so junior…all the time."

"Junior in some ways, but senior in so many others…at three in the morning you are the most accessible doctor on the wards. First contact. It's a massive responsibility. With that responsibility comes respect."

"Really. I don't feel it."

"It comes."

"If there was respect they wouldn't have done an incident form."

"No. You're taking it the wrong way, personally. The incident form is irrelevant. It wasn't a judgment on you, it was an observation that when a fast bleep was put out the doctor couldn't come because he was doing something else. So what? If you can accept that now and again, purely by virtue of the fact that you see so many patients, you are bound to be involved in a complaint or an incident form, you will be able to work naturally, learn, and progress. If you can accept that you work within a network of continuous feedback, but without having your outlook obscured by it, you will achieve whatever you want to achieve."

"You make it sound almost cosy. It isn't. In the middle of the night I get shouted at if I don't come. And relatives write down what I'm saying as though everything is a statement."

"Well…so might you when you have a relative in hospital. Are you coming back to work next week?"

" I haven't decided."

"That's OK, take your time."

The silent patient

I hear you

I heard all of this yesterday, but I doubt anyone will ever know because I am dying. They didn't think I was listening, but listening is about all I can do. Perhaps one day there will be a way of reading these final thoughts, some scan, some process. I hope so, because they need to know.

I was reasonably alert when I came into hospital, but as the pneumonia progressed I grew more and more drowsy. When I lapsed into this coma – I suppose that's how you describe it - they called a doctor to see me. I heard it all.

The nurse rushed away from me – her shoes squeaked into the distance – and called over to a colleague,

"Bed 9 looks awful, her saturations are 78 percent."

"Put her on a non-rebreather…turn the oxygen right up…" answered the other.

"She's scoring 9 though, should I put out a call?"

"Yes. No. Let's take a look at her…"

I heard her feet settle at the end of my bed. She picked up my wrist and called out, "Bleep the on-call, I think the saturations are under-reading because she's shut down."

Fifteen minutes later a doctor arrived.

"How is she?"

"Like we said. Drowsy, shut down. I would have put out an emergency call if I knew you were going to take this long…"

"Sorry, I had three others to see first."

He was gentle, and spoke to me as he examined me. He summoned his senior because he was worried, and they talked to one another by the bed. It was strange – he must have thought I could hear if he talked to me during the examination, but if he thought I could hear why did he talk *about* me, in pretty impersonal terms, so close to the bed? The senior one spoke first,

"She's going off. Type 2 respiratory failure. Is she for escalation or ward based care?"

"It doesn't say she's not in the notes."

"OK, then we should take her to HDU."

"For non-invasive?"

"Not right away, but for an arterial line, monitoring…"

"Can I do the line."

"How many have you done?"

"She would be my fifth."

"How did the other four go?"

"I missed one."

"Ok, you can do it, she's got a decent radial artery."

He paused,

"I'm just thinking…if she should be for…"

"For what?"

"Everything. Let me just look at the x-ray and read the notes again. I mean, the ceiling will be non-invasive ventilation, ITU won't take her…"

"She's not that old."

"It's not that. It says here that her exercise tolerance is usually 30 yards," (that's true, my lungs have been awful for years due to smoking) "…and she was being assessed for home oxygen three months ago. She's close to end stage. Let's talk over here."

They moved away. How very sensitive! They talked quietly at the nurse's station, I think (I didn't have the strength to open my eyes) - too quietly for me to hear - but I know they were deciding if I should 'get everything' or not. If I should be given a chance to live. Why move away now?

Then I realised what they were doing. They were trying to be decent, observing a social convention. I don't think they were really taking my possible feelings into account, because if my feelings were really uppermost in their minds they wouldn't have even started to have the conversation in front of me. I mean, what do I care how many bloody 'lines' that doctor has inserted? They forgot themselves, and it suddenly dawned on them that it was not the done thing to speak so frankly in the presence of a dying woman. They glanced at my face, probably, and wondered – oh God, what if she can hear? - and they became uncomfortable. I've seen and heard a lot of that here; behaviours that are explained not by the needs of the patients, but by the sensibilities of the doctors and nurses.

Anyway, I'm still here, same bed, same ward. Evidently it wasn't felt to be in my interests to be carted along the corroder and attached to a machine. My family came in and spoke to me, then to the doctors, and they talked some more in a relatives' room. They spoke *for* me. Quite right too. Later on I heard a nurse say they had *'agreed not for resus.'* Fair enough. If these final moments of reflection come to a sudden stop I don't want them running in and having a go at me. But I didn't really need to hear all the explication, the justification, the gloomy prophecy bandied about with indifference. If you read this, medical people, be more careful with what you say in future. It takes very little energy to listen, and the words go in.

*

Comment I do not write this from a position of moral superiority. I have said many of those things, and worse, next to unconscious patients. It is expedient and, dare I say it, sometimes necessary to have clinically brutal conversations with colleagues in close proximity to obtunded, delirious, encephalopathic or comatose patients, especially in emergencies. But it's worth reflecting that we have very little idea as to how much they can hear. Some will be just starting to deteriorate, and their faculties will be reasonably well preserved. Others will be truly insensible. The safest policy is strict separation from the bedside, but we are unlikely ever to adhere to that. So how does this fantasy help? If nothing else, it reminds us that behind every impassive exterior there is a mind, and that mind might, *might*, be as alert as yours.

Don't tell me the odds

I survived the war…the odds were long for prisoners like me, but I managed it. Luck played a part, but so did resilience, and, though it I can't prove it, my 'survival gene'. I won't tell you exactly what I went through but I was in Singapore when it fell in 1942, I was captured and imprisoned, and I was starved. I saw friends and fellow soldiers swell with malnutrition, vitamin deficiencies and heart failure, and a good number fell to the ground on the building works. There was cruelty. The chances were that I would not survive, but I did.

Since that time I have dodged a few bullets: a car accident on the M1 in 1975 ('a miracle you survived' said the intensive care nurse when I came back to thank them for all they had done), and the bad bout of influenza in '92 nearly did for me. I was on a ventilator for two weeks, and developed kidney failure as well. The family were brought in, and they heard that I was 'very, very unlikely' to survive. But I did. I'm a survivor.

So now I come to this week. I've not been right for months, but 5 days ago I got properly sick. It looks like the heart is catching up with me because suddenly, just like the chaps in the prison camp with wet beriberi, my legs started swelling and I got desperately short of breath. Apparently my chest x-ray shows that my heart is hugely enlarged, and after the echo test I overheard someone say that it was pumping like an old carrier bag. I get the meaning. I've got bad heart failure, from the fags I'm sure, and two of the valves are shot. But I'm what…born in '24…I'm just shy of 90, I've done pretty well.

So one of the random doctors came along this morning and did the usual checks, crossed some things off the drug chart and added some more, then looked at me, all sensitive in the eyes, and sat on the bed. He said,

"Eric, I'd like to ask you something that you may not have thought about before."

"Yes."

"It's about what we should do if your heart were to suddenly stop. If you were to have a heart attack, a cardiac arrest."

"I know what you mean. But I haven't thought about it."

"As you might know, we often call the emergency team to try to restart hearts with chest compressions or electric shocks, but we have to be sure that there is a good chance that it will work. Sometimes, if the heart is already very weak, the chance of it working is very small indeed, and the damage that those attempts can do is quite significant."

"So what are you saying?"

"Well, in your case, I don't think it would be a good idea. We know your heart has become very weak over the last few years, without you knowing it, and if it were to stop – and I'm not anticipating that it will, you're quite stable – the chance of getting it going again, strongly enough for you wake up and be close to how you are now, is unlikely."

"How unlikely?"

"I can't give you a definite number."

"Don't they know?"

"Well, I did read a study that found for every 30 people in their nineties who were resuscitated only 1 left the hospital. But everyone is different, it's a decision that needs to be made on an individual basis."

"But from where you're standing the odds are bad."

"Yes."

I really hadn't considered all this before. Perhaps I should have. You see, I enjoy my life, and I have confidence in my ability to survive. I've proven it, after all, time and again. But yes, I am older now, the floppy bag in my chest is on its last set of batteries, so I suppose I need to listen. But I wasn't prepared to say – 'OK, mark me down for no resuscitation.' I'm sure it's awful, being compressed and shocked, I'm sure the machines you have to go on are uncomfortable, but I've had worse. They way he spoke, I'm not sure he'll agree to put me down for resuscitation anyway, it sounds like it's his decision. But he did ask me. Didn't he? Or did he tell me. I don't know. So I've left it for now. I want to think about it.

The doctor sits in the canteen with his team. His junior colleague asks,

"So, the old chap with the bad heart. Do I do a DNAR form?"

The senior doctor replies,

"Tricky, tricky. In my opinion he has next to zero chance of surviving a crash call. I made that pretty clear didn't I, within the bounds of compassion."

"I think so."

"Would you give chemotherapy to a cancer patient if there was, say, a 2% chance of it working?"

"No, of course not."

"In fact, you wouldn't even discuss it. It wouldn't be on the agenda. So you could argue, why are we even discussing resuscitation with this man? Statistically, medically, it's an irrelevance. It won't work."

"You don't know that. And you're talking about the end of his life. The moment of death. He's bound to have an opinion. You didn't say it was guaranteed *not* to work."

"Trust me, it won't. He might get a pulse back but he wouldn't get off inotropes afterwards. And his kidneys are already working at 20% capacity. They will fail too. And will intensive care take him? No. If he stays for resus we're holding out a false hope. It's dishonest."

"So I should do the form shouldn't I? It's the weekend, we can't leave it."

"I'll need to go back to him, see if he agrees. He wanted more time, so be it."

Back on the ward.

"Hello again Eric."

"Hello."

"I wondered if you had thought any more about our conversation."

He sat down again, carefully addressed the subject. He made a good case. And you know what I said? Well, I didn't say much. I didn't have the energy. I couldn't be bothered to tell this doctor about my scrapes with death, about the commitment I made to myself back in '42 *never* to give in, *never* to accept fate without a fight…because that's what got me through it, and that's what got me off the ventilator in '92. It was survivability. I'm still the same man, mentally, if not physically. Call me stubborn, but his statistics don't apply to me. I've proved that. I'm going for it.

The doctors' mess

"Did he agree?" asks the junior.

"No."

"What do we do?"

"Respect it."

"It's crazy…it's not the right decision?"

"Well I'm not signing it."

"I'll talk to him some more. Do you mind if I try?"

"And coerce him?"

"Persuade him."

"He's made up his mind. It's not a rational thing. It's about not letting go of 90 years of life without an argument. I understand it. I don't agree, but I understand."

"And if he arrests, we'll look pretty silly, leaving a 90 year old with severe heart disease for resuscitation."

"So be it."

Signs

Another brief exercise in wondering what it's like for patients who meet our kind in certain situations.

The other day a junior colleague described to me, over lunch, a patient who had been admitted with unusual and florid signs, due to a disease that is not commonly seen. I clapped my hands and said, 'Excellent!' And then I heard myself, and was embarrassed. The signs indicated advanced disease, but the prospect of seeing them excited me as a clinician. In that staff canteen, far away from the patient, I could show my appreciation for signs that made the patient a sure source of learning for our trainees, and a jolt to the enthusiasm that once motivated my own nervous forays onto the wards as a third year student.

oOo

(From a hospital diary)

I had an inkling, but when I saw him coming I smiled, as I do to any who approach my bed. His eyes darted from my face to my hands (where the rash is) to my abdomen, which was completely hidden beneath the sheet anyway. He must have been told about me. I had overheard a small gaggle of students discussing an imminent teaching session which was due to begin at 11. And time was now pressing, for it was ten to 11. He introduced himself, asked me how I was, and came straight out with it –

"I wondered if you'd mind if I bought a few students along to ask you some questions and...examine you." I said nothing. It's happened before. But he was determined. "Just a handful. Is that OK?" It was clearly important to him.

I would rather not have. I mean, what was in it for me? It wasn't the fear of being made uncomfortable, but I was quite happy reading my book, temporarily escaping my dismal fate. The pleasure of 'being taught on', if there was one, would be in observing the revelatory expressions on the students' faces as they felt organs they had not felt before, or as they recognised lesions that they had only read about in books. But really, I have my own worries, and the education of our future doctors is not one of them.

"It's alright." I said, though it wasn't. I had a duty to be helpful, and he had a duty to press me, for the sake of his students. I suppose.

30 minutes later.

They were very nice, each one of them. And the consultant tried to make sure they didn't hurt me, though one of them did by pressing on my liver like a novice baker kneading dough. Just one thing though: one of the young woman stood up from bending over to get a close look at the rash, and said,

"It's not classic."

Well, sorry! I'll try to develop it, rub it up into a proper horror! My feedback to you - *never*, say *anything* negative about another person's body, even if it is diseased. Isn't that a basic social skill? But otherwise, no complaints, except for the fact that for all the sense of reward and betterment in the young faces, the fact remains that the 'learning points' would not be there unless I was ill. And I am *very* ill.

A day later.

A new admission, into the bed next door. She looks interesting, but sick - bright yellow all over. The teaching doctor came along a couple of hours ago. He glanced at me as he passed, nodded and smiled. No words. He doesn't need me now. And he approached my new neighbour, and said, after the pleasantries,

"I wondered if you'd mind if I bought a few students along to ask you some questions and…examine you. Just a handful. Is that OK?"

The cheek.

The apprenticeship

Fade to green

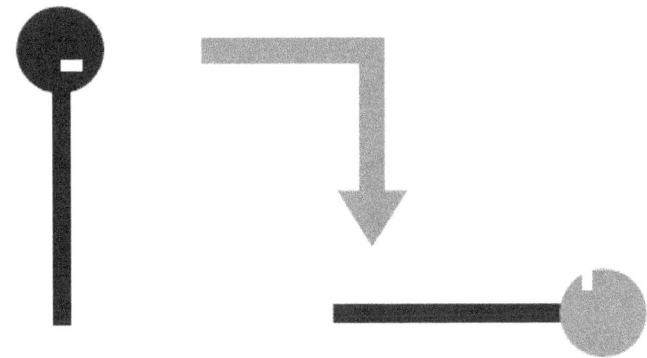

I fainted half a dozen times during my training. It's a problem that worries quite a few people, so here are some of my fainting tales. They may make you feel better.

I should have known it would be a problem because during GCSE biology I was asked to dissect a cow's eye. It slipped and rolled under my scalpel, glancing at me as it turned. My teacher asked me if I was alright. Apparently I had gone green. As soon as he said that I began to feel green. I lay my head down on the cool workbench and soon recovered. It was close one.

Then, before applying to med school, I spent a night in the local Casualty department. I watched a junior doctor try to prise a splinter from the hand of a young lady. It was hurting her, and she kept yelping. The doctor got irritated and said the anaesthetic 'should be working'. He kept digging into her hand, she started to cry, I felt lightheaded, moved my legs to keep the blood flowing…and I was out. It wasn't the gore, it was the negative emotion – I think. Anyway, they put me on a trolley, checked my blood glucose, and the same doctor told me the only explanation for such low levels was an insulinoma. I got home, looked it up, and for some months assumed there was something unpleasant growing within me.

So to med school, and the post-mortem. I had been really looking forward to this. The Professor of pathology lifted out a series of pre-mobilised organs and held them up for those of us in the viewing gallery to see. I glanced past his gloved hands at the cadaver, glimpsed the head, saw the juices drip off the liver...and down I went. As usual I came around immediately, to be told that when the Professor heard the thump he looked up and called out, 'Will someone see if she's alright?'

Then came venesection practise. My partner shakily inserted a needle into one side of my elbow vein and out the other, causing a 'sixer' sized haematoma. As it swelled I began to sweat, the edges of my visual field closed in and I immediately sat on the floor with my head between my knees. Another close one. However, come the first day of my third year as a medical student, entering the wards at last after two years of lectures, I did less well. We met the house officer (she seemed so grown up) and were told that it was our job to do the phlebotomy rounds each morning. She assembled a vacutainer set and asked me to roll my sleeve up. Pretending to take blood, she held the needle a centimetre from my skin. My brain said NO WAY, the sweat came on and clunk, I was down. The clunk was the sound of my forehead connecting with the edge of a sink. The rest of the day went fine, but the bruise took a week to settle.

I entered the operating theatre as a student on a vascular surgical firm with great trepidation. For some reason the blood and gore did not affect me as it did some others. I watched a consultant repair a ruptured abdominal aneurysm, observed the blood as it pour off the table into his white rubber boots, saw him curse as he nicked the spleen and was forced to remove it...but the fascination allowed no room for vasovagal syncope.

But I was not cured. For my elective I travelled to Nepal via Delhi. In a busy Indian market square I asked a cobbler to repair the soles of my shoes. He stuck strips of orange rubber onto them with stringy glue that he applied with a stick. His friend tried to clean out my ears with a cotton bud while I waited, but I pushed him away. I was pleased with the job on the shoes though. Anyway, come the first day on the wards in Kathmandu I was feeling a bit rough, having accidentally swallowed some tap water while shaving two days before. I stood in the breeze of an inadequate fan, watched a cat slink between the legs of a hospital bed and lick some organic fluid from the edge of bucket containing sharps...and there we go! I came to on a bed with ECG stickers on my chest. The Professor, a very serious man, asked me if I had a heart problem. I said no. What really upset me was the group of students and doctors at the foot of the bed peering at the soles of my shoes.

After that there were no more uncontrolled total faints. I came close during a stressful central line insertion as a senior house officer, but I think a hangover predisposed me to it. I slipped to the floor, put my cheek to the plastic tiles, sweating, the wire still sticking out of the patient's neck, and fought it until a nurse brought a cup of ice cold water. Within minutes I was back on my feet, hands clean, fresh gloves on, ready to finish the job. I don't think the patient ever knew what was going on.

Since then I have found myself in many faint-prone situations, but I am glad to report that it is no longer a problem. Blood, stress, chaos, suffering…none of it hits my pulse rate or blood pressure. Rest assured, if you are a fainter, it gets better.

The moment: a tale of three doctors

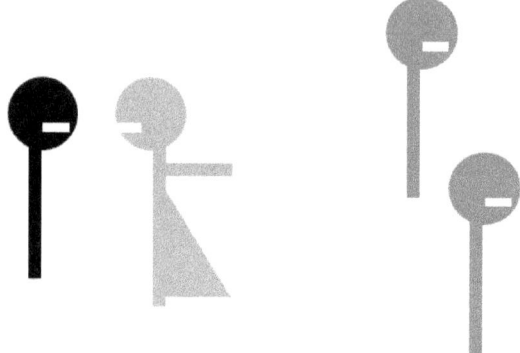

'...in the raw cold of that leaden crisis in the four-and-twenty hours when the vital force of all the noblest and prettiest things that live is at its lowest...'

Charles Dickens, Our Mutual Friend

―――

'This seraph-band, each waved his hand:

It was a heavenly, sight!

They stood as signals to the land,

Each one a lovely light'

Samuel Taylor Coleridge, The Rime of the Ancient Mariner

oOo

3.45AM A medical ward

Mark Smithson, two years qualified, held the telephone to his ear and spoke urgently, trying hard not to impart his sense of desperation.

"I am really worried about him. His blood pressure is much lower than earlier, I can't give him more diuretic, but his breathing needs it."

"From what you've told me there's nothing more to be done at the moment. Isn't he end stage?"

"I don't think so, he only had his heart attack four months ago. There's something about him I don't understand. Can you come and see him?"

"Look, it's pretty clear what the problem is. His heart failure is getting worse, perhaps he's been run a bit dry as well. Give a few boluses of fluid, see how he responds."

"When will you be free? There's something about him…"

"Why don't you let me know how it looks in a couple of hours, and if he is no better I'll come and see him. It's a really busy down here. I think you can manage the situation. Are you okay with that?"

"Yes." But Mark meant No.

He began to put the phone down. He was deeply tired, working the third of five night shifts and not yet adjusted to the nocturnal rhythm. His tongue was thick with cheap, over-concentrated coffee. The battle, one of many, could not be won right now.

He heard a rasping breath by his ear, and looked up. An old man in a hospital gown, a patient whom Mark did not recognize, stood by his side. He placed a cold grey-veined hand on Mark's wrist and held it.

"Excuse me! Err...sir, do you want go back to your bed?"

"Shhh! They're sleeping."

"What are you doing?"

"You can ask me later. This is your moment. I am your moment. I'm here to show you what happens."

"What happens to what?"

"What happens to you if you put that phone down. Come with me."

The old man took away his hand and beckoned. Mark stood and followed, completely in his power. Looking back he saw that the phone's beige handset hovered in the air above the nurses' station; he had forgotten to replace it. The two of them, one short and bowed, the other tall and young, left the ward (there were no nurses to observe them - where had they gone?) and entered a corridor. A blue light bathed the floor, and Mark looked up to see what had happened to the lighting.

"Look through this door Mark." A door had appeared in what had previously been an exterior wall.

He peered through a small rectangular aperture, into what should have been the night air; instead he saw a gleaming new department. A patient was being wheeled through an ante room toward what looked like the doors of an operating theatre.

"What is this?"

"Look at the anaesthetist Mark. I give you the gift of lip reading for now."

"What's that thing moving over the patient?" A large white disc, the size of a dustbin lid, emitting the same blue light that Mark had already noted, hung from a gantry.

"That's just a gamma bath. Patients are routinely sterilised in 2029, there's global antibiotic resistance. You can't do an operation if there are any microbes on the skin. The surgeon is under her own gamma shower, round the back. It doesn't seem to cause any damage over a career, that's what they are told. Can you hear what he's saying, the anaesthetist?"

Mark focused on the man's lips and found that he could understand everything. The anaesthetist was chatting to a younger colleague.

"Sounds complicated."

"Who should I refer her to?"

"I'd suggest Dr Smithson."

"I've heard he's…"

"He can be a bit difficult sometimes. Once he get's a bee in his bonnet he jumps up and down if he doesn't get his own way. It doesn't make him a lot of friends, but for someone in your patient's situation I think he's the one I'd choose. He doesn't give up, he doesn't mind causing a few ripples."

"I heard he was a bit of a nightmare. You can't run around demanding the whole hospital does what you want. There are other patients, other consultants. I heard he refuses to give up on anybody, even when the writing is on the wall."

"Perhaps he over-treats sometimes, but the fact is he's probably the one you'd want looking after *your* mother, father, whoever..."

Mark felt the cold hand on his shoulder, a finger brushing his neck.

"That's enough."

"They were talking about me. They used my surname."

"So they were. Now come with me, I've got something else to show you."

They walked to the end of the corridor until they came to another door. Mark looked through another small window, and saw that the door was connected to the back of an outpatient clinic room. He saw the back of his own, more aged head. A patient faced his older self, seemingly unaware of the younger doctor observing the consultation.

"So there's nothing more you can do doctor?"

"I can't see any other options. I'm sorry."

"So that's it. I've got to live with this. Or not live, if it gets worse."

"I'll write to your GP, explain it all."

"But she can't help me. I need you to write to them, get them to agree to fund the nano-stems."

"It's not my decision, it's been agreed that patients with renal failure don't qualify…heart, brain, liver failure yes, but not kidney, not yet."

"But since the ban on anti-rejection drugs there's no hope of a transplant, stems are my only option now. You're sentencing me to death!"

"Not me. We don't agree with it, but we can't overturn that decision. I'm sorry. Things might change, I'll keep an open appointment on the system…"

"Right. Right. I get it." The patient left. And now Mark's point of view followed the patient, he flew through the room and into the waiting area, leaving his older self behind. He saw the patient sit down heavily, heard him sigh sadly. Mark watched him as he typed a message to his partner - 'No luck.' A nurse came to ask the patient if he was alright, she seemed to know him.

"Final decision?" she asked.

"Seems like it."

"I shouldn't say this…but have you thought going to see someone else. There's a consultant at St. Jude's, he's managed to get stems for a few patients off protocol. He just keeps writing letters until they agree…"

The patient left, thanking her politely, not really taking in the advice. Then the nurse walked up to a colleague, and whispered,

"It's a shame. They *can* get them, if they fight for it. He doesn't care, or can't be bothered, if you ask me…he doesn't exactly put himself out does he…"

The scene shrank away as Mark felt himself fly back through the small window into the corridor. His scrawny guide was already walking back to the ward, and Mark hurried to catch up with him. They re-entered the ward. The old man walked resolutely to his bed, leant over stiffly to reach the edge of a sheet, drew the linen back and folded his wasted legs into the uninviting space beneath. He lay back, his eyes closed, but spoke again,

"Those are your futures. Now go back to the phone, but before you hang up think hard. Your registrar is still listening."

"I don't understand."

"You have a choice. What does your patient need, *right* now?"

"Someone who knows more medicine than me to work out what's going on."

"And what's stopping you *insisting* on that senior review?"

"I asked didn't I? And I got some advice. What more can I do?"

"What would you do if it was your father?"

"I'd insist."

"But not for this patient? Why?"

"I...I don't want to annoy my registrar, he's busy."

"So it's *you* you're worried about. Reputation. Ripples. Goodnight." He rolled onto his side.

Mark's hand encircled the static, hovering handset. Time restarted. A nurse walked past briskly, a buzzer sounded, a patient groaned in her sleep and asked for her long dead husband.

"No...wait!" Mark's voice, stern, assertive.

"What?"

"I need you to come to see him. He is deteriorating quickly, I don't know what's wrong with him. Sorry, I've tried, but I need you to see him *now*. It can't wait."

"I...I...told you, I'm stuck here..."

"Shall I call the consultant at home?"

"What?! Christ, you mean it don't you. OK, OK, I'm coming."

Mark could only imagine what he was saying under his breath.

When the registrar arrived Mark nodded, embarrassed, and led him straight to the patient. His bed was opposite that of the spectral guide. Mark glanced at it, and saw that it was now empty, in fact it was neatly made in readiness for a new patient. The registrar assessed the cardiac patient, scrutinised the ECG and began to smile.

"Very strange. Normal saturations, but this ECG is different. Right heart strain. He needs a scan urgently, he may have a pulmonary embolism. And if we're right I'd be tempted to thrombolyse him. Nice one!"

"Well we don't know yet."

"It's likely, he's been in bed for two weeks with those huge swollen legs."

"Thank you, for coming."

"You knew it wasn't right. That's the lesson I'd take away from this - believe in your instincts...and persist! But you don't need to learn that lesson, it seems."

The registrar left Mark to make the arrangements for the scan. Mark returned to his ailing cardiac patient and looked over once again toward the empty bed. There was somebody in it. A bony hand beckoned him over.

"Good decision Dr Smithson."

"Thank you."

"You alright doc?" A nurse looked at him quizzically. "Too many night shifts, talking to yourself?"

"I'm fine. I'm fine."

Mark thought he could discern a faint blue glow beneath the sheet, but the morning sun soon banished the impression.

oOo

With apologies to Dr Who (The Day of the Doctor) and Dickens' A Christmas Carol

Fate night

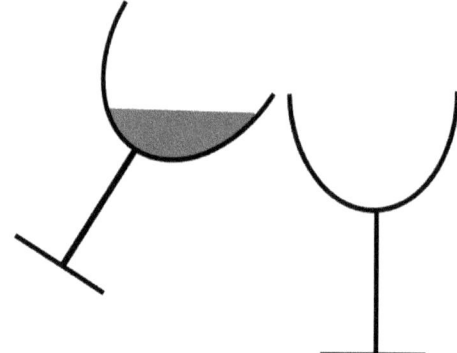

Here is a tale that examines medical motivation, duty, sacrifice and the source of a doctor's job satisfaction. It is inspired by a number of experiences, but the medical scenario is fictional.

An intravenous drug user, Sally, is transferred to the ward from Casualty. The ward doctor, Elaine, reads the notes: 'diagnosis – sepsis, ?source.' Antibiotics have been prescribed, the chest x-ray is said to be normal (Elaine is not so sure when she looks at it), the urine is clear, and there are no obvious signs of heart valve infection. It's 4.30pm, and although Elaine shouldn't really have to re-examine Sally so soon after the transfer, she does, just to make sure she's alright. And she is definitely *not* alright. She looks nothing like the patient described by the nurse who provided the handover. Sally is drowsy, her heart is racing, she seems breathless. Elaine calls her registrar for advice, but he is stuck in clinic. Elaine works through the problem, and wonders whether one of Sally's heart valves is infected after all. It is common for bacteria to travel through the veins into which heroine is injected, up to the heart, where they can settle and multiply, eating into the fragile leaflets of tissue.

What Elaine doesn't mention to the registrar is that she has a date with her boyfriend tonight. It's her anniversary, and they have a table booked for 8pm.

Elaine spends the next hour trying to correct Sally's sagging blood pressure by prescribing fluids, then correcting her low oxygen levels by turning up the oxygen supply. She calls a cardiologist, and she agrees that an echocardiogram is indicated urgently. She, the cardiologist, is happy to do it after her clinic, probably around 6.15pm.

"Should I move her to intensive care?" asks Elaine.

"Get them to review her, but at the moment we don't know which way she is going – it could still just be a bad urine infection after all, she might pick up later."

Elaine calls intensive care and the outreach team give their assessment – the patient does not yet require transfer, await the result of the echo.

The echocardiogram, performed at 6.45pm, proves that one of the heart valves is leaking badly. It doesn't identify a vegetation (a lump of bacteria sitting on the valve), but given the context of sepsis and drug use, it's a fair bet that Sally has endocarditis.

"Is she worse now compared to when she came in?" asks the cardiologist.

"I guess so, because they didn't tell us she looked this sick when they arranged the transfer to the ward. What's going to happen now?"

"It depends. If the antibiotics don't stabilise the situation and the valve continues to be destroyed, she may need a valve replacement."

"As an emergency."

"Errr yes. Don't you think!" The tone is sarcastic. Elaine shuts up for a minute. She hasn't seen this before. She watches as the cardiologist packs up the echo machine, then asks,

"What now then? Do you want me to do anything?"

"Well I think she needs to be in intensive care. Can you get them back, tell them what the diagnosis is...I'll call the consultant myself when I've put this machine away." It's 7.15. Elaine texts her boyfriend.

The intensive care team agree that Sally needs to come round, but the bed is not yet ready. It will be another 2 hours. But the transfer is precautionary, she won't come to harm from the delay

"She needs a central line." says the registrar, "I can do it now-ish, before she goes round. I'll do it in theatres. I've got another urgent review to do first...can you go to theatres and book it in?" Elaine nods, and hesitates by the door of the ward. This seems a good time to hand over to the late team. As she begins to bleep the on-call SHO a nurse runs up to her,

"She's unrousable. I think it might be the Heroine, but she can't have had any here. Her pupils are tiny. Can you see her?" Elaine hurries to Sally's bed, and agrees. She asks for some Naloxone, the antidote to Heroine. The drug perks her up. But the underlying problem, the valve, is unchanged. A phone goes off, a nurse answers,

"Elaine, it's theatres, they're ready for the central line but you need to book it in before they call for the patient..."

Elaine hurries to theatres. She meets her registrar in the corridor. He asks what's happening, and Elaine explains everything. Then, at then end, she says,

"I'm really sorry to throw this in...but I've got to get away for something."

"When?"

"Well, half an hour ago."

"What still needs to be done?"

"Booking this central line in, and handing over."

"Look, I'll book it in, you hand over, then go. Intensive care will take it form there."

Elaine is on the phone to the on-call doctor when her bleep goes off.

"Give us a minute, I'll call you back on your extension." she says to the on-call, then answers the bleep. It's the intensive care registrar,

"You didn't tell me her clotting was all off. She needs fresh frozen plasma, or I can't do this central line. Can you organise it...right now?" And he hangs up. There is no conversation. Elaine gets back to the on-call, but the on-call is desperate to get back to a case in the resuscitation bay. Elaine must order the blood herself. She glances at her watch – it's 7.55pm.

She blinks back a tear. It was an important night…that's all. It takes fifteen minutes to organise plasma. Then she prepares, finally, to go. A nurse approaches. Elaine avoids eye contact, but it's absurd, she knows the nurse, and knows what it is about.

"Elaine….Sally's sister has just arrived."

"OK. OK. Give me a minute."

Elaine calls her boyfriend. He is in the restaurant. Elaine reckons on fifteen minutes with the sister, to explain everything, then another forty to get to the restaurant. The evening is not yet finished.

Sally's sister tells Elaine that there are two children, one in care, one still at home. She places a photo of the younger child on the bedside cabinet. Elaine looks at it, and wonders why someone so innocent, this two year old girl, should lose a mother to such a disease, a complication of addiction. Elaine feels a surge of warmth towards Sally, and chastises herself for worrying so much about her own concerns, the petty matters of her comfortable life. But still, it would be nice to get out of here now.

The handover is complete. The last remaining ties to the hospital, to Sally, are severed. Elaine has her coat on. It is 8.40pm. Her bleep goes off again, but it's an outside line - 'friendly fire' as they say. Only friends and family, in general, know what name or bleep number to ask for through the switchboard.

"Hi, it's Elaine!" she says, when the phone connection has been made.

"Ah, hello there. My name is David Banbury. I'm the cardiothoracic registrar on call at St. Thomas's. We had a call from one of your cardiologists earlier to say there may be a patient who needs an emergency transfer. Can you give me an update?"

"Well, she's going to intensive care."

"I know. But I need to know how she is now, so we can arrange to get her over before she collapses completely. What's her BP, pulse, renal function…What's the history?"

"I…I don't know all that."

"Well can you find out?"

"…"

"Hello?"

"Yes. I can find out. How can I get hold of you?"

"I'll give you my mobile. Are you on call?"

"No. I've stayed late."

"Well I'm sorry. But this patient has one chance, and a small one at that if what I have heard so far is true. You seem to be the only doctor around who knows anything about her. Your cardiologist wasn't even sure of the name!"

Ninety minutes later Elaine drive straight home. Her boyfriend has called to say he is leaving the restaurant, and he is waiting for her as she comes through the front door of their flat. She explains, he listens, as he always does. He understands why it was so important that she stayed, but makes the point that this evening was their *third* attempt to eat out together. The anniversary had actually been six weeks ago.

"It won't always be like this." says Elaine. He nods, but the look in his eyes suggests to her that we isn't so sure…about anything.

"Well I hope she's grateful." is all he can add.

6 weeks later.

Sally is transferred back from the cardiothoracic unit. Her stay there has been a rocky one. Before the valve operation she arrested twice, and she remained on their intensive care unit for four weeks with complications, chest drains, resistant organisms, the lot. But now she is back. And not only that, she has been sent back to Elaine's ward. She needs a side room because of the multi-resistant bacteria that now reside on her skin. Elaine is actually quite excited. She knows that she played an important role in Sally's management…not crucial, not technical, not heroic, but important. She helped bring the major decision makers together on the night in question, and her clear reports, her calm referrals, ensured that the clinical scenario was accurately communicated and acted upon.

"Hello Sally." says Elaine, on the ward round.

"Who are you?" asks Sally.

"Elaine, one of your doctors."

"Well doctor, can you sort this f****** place out, they said I could have a telly in here but I still haven't got one…"

The eyes and the ears: why Adam blew the whistle

Previously I wrote a [dialogue between two junior doctors](). They discussed why Michael would not report, to some higher authority, the dangerous incompetence of a consultant. In this second dialogue, Adam explains to his friend why he [phoned the GMC]() to report dangerous staffing levels. This dialogue seeks to illustrate why a doctor might feel compelled to act, rather than just watch, shake their head and move on.

This is imaginary, obviously. It is intended to describe the thoughts that a whistle blower might have.

Adam and his friend sit in a beer garden. Adam occasionally looks over his shoulder to check who has taken the adjacent table.

"Was it you?" asks Adam's friend.

"What?"

"Who called the GMC."

"What did you hear?"

"That someone blew the whistle on A and E."

"What else did you hear?"

"That it was about staffing levels, lack of support...it *was* you wasn't it?"

"Why do you think it was me?"

"Because you've been going on about it for ages."

"That's the point I guess. I wasn't seeing any changes at all. I was out of ideas."

"So did you actually complain first, officially...through proper channels?"

"I told the clinical lead that I thought we were too thin on the ground. Several times."

"And what did she say?"

"That it 'will get better'. That 'when the deanery send us more juniors we'll be fine'. Mañana, mañana."

"Did you have examples, of poor staffing leading to bad outcomes?"

"How can you get that evidence? We're working on the ground, struggling, we work our arses off to keep the ship afloat, some people die, most don't, how do I know if any particular death is directly related to not enough staff? How do I know if our department has got more deaths or delayed diagnoses that average? I don't have that overview."

"So how can you justify blowing the whistle? You don't know that the department was actually under-performing."

"If you follow that line of reasoning, no-one would ever stand up and say anything, they would have no confidence in their own opinion. *'I'm just a cog in a machine, I'm not driving the machine'*. To justify NOT saying anything you have to have complete faith in the driver. Do I have faith in the driver? I don't know, I don't know the people who run the hospital . All I know is that sometimes it's hell in that department and patients are falling off their chairs in the waiting room."

"And despite not *knowing*, you made the call. Where did you develop that confidence in yourself?"

"It's not confidence. It didn't come easy. I waited for months and months before making that phone call. Nearly a year in fact. But nothing was changing."

"It has now."

"I know."

"You should feel proud."

"I don't. I just feel sick when I walk through A and E. At least staff move through it so quickly the current set of juniors don't recognize me as the troublemaker. The consultants do. But a few have told me that they are pleased I did it."

"Weren't they embarrassed?"

"No, I don't think so. They thought the same as me. When someone actually does it…does something positive, everyone suddenly says 'Yeah, I agree, it's unacceptable…'. Like the emperor's new clothes, everyone pretends it's fine, they can manage, then someone pipes up and the truth becomes clear to all, undeniable. Weird psychology."

"But why did it take your call? The Trust knew about the situation, the department was aware...not just from your comments...but it took the fear of a GMC investigation to do anything."

"I honestly don't know."

"Has anyone from senior management spoken to you?"

"Yep."

"And...?"

"It was all very reasonable, understanding, respectful in fact."

"Fake?"

"Actually no. We got into a good discussion. He made me feel relaxed, and we went into it in some detail."

"Such as?"

"The bigger picture. He allowed me to push him...to draw him out...to reveal HIS thoughts about whistleblowing. It wasn't the greatest example of whisteblowing in history was it, really, more of an alert I think…so I don't think he minded talking about it. So we got into the bigger picture. He encouraged me to think about scale, to think about the hospital as a unit, providing care to all of its patients and to the whole community. Elective and emergency.

Babies, kids...not just the sort of patient *I* was seeing. Those in charge have to decide where to put the resources, where to place the staff..."

"So only *they* have the overview, and the knowledge..."

"Perhaps, but it went further. I said yeah, you have to make hard decisions, to ration basically, but you in turn are being rationed, by the government, who have demanded that you save x million this year as a share of the £20 billion of efficiency savings. He liked that."

"He didn't really agree to pass the buck onto the government did he?"

"Not as such. But perhaps he should have. I might have sympathised with him."

"You can take the bigger picture further you know Adam."

"How?"

"To society as a whole. Why does the government demand we save £20 billion?"

"Because the economy is screwed. Austerity."

"Yes, that's the environment we live in. But within that environment the government has decided to squeeze the health service because it has a duty to maintain other parts of the state at the same time. Defence, social security, prisons...so in their eyes, the bigger picture demands that Trusts feel the pain. That's the price of austerity, of long term economic stability. We don't have that overview, the *really* big overview."

"You really believe that? No wonder *you* didn't make that call. You've intellectualised it to death."

"Perhaps."

"I said I sympathized with the big picture, but ultimately it doesn't cut it. Because it's not *our* business to care about the bigger picture, don't you see? Resources are be sent down according to the best judgements or intentions of our political masters, or moved around the Trust by our senior managers, but we must concern ourselves with what the effect of those decisions is at ground level."

"Humour me a minute Adam, I'm not criticising you…but *why* whinge about those decisions? We *live* in the big picture. We are citizens in a democracy, we, as a society, voted for austerity and hardship. We ARE cogs. That's the state we're in, we should just do our best within it. "

"It doesn't matter. We, as doctors, work in a *small* world, the hospital…and we are there to make patients better. *We* are the ones with the eyes and the ears to tell the ones who move those resources around that their decisions are proving destructive. *We* are the ones who must tell them if minimum acceptable standards are not being maintained. Who else is going to spot that? If not us, who?"

"But doesn't everyone think that their little domain is under resourced, straining to maintain minimum standards? We can't have all of them ringing the GMC helpline."

"I agree. And that's why it took me a year. I challenged myself over and over again, told myself it was just me, just a bad run of shifts, that my seniors had recognised the problem and were dealing with it…but nothing happened! So I did it. I reassured myself that it was up to me to tell them that here, in this case, the balance wasn't right."

"Eyes and ears."

"Yep. That's what Francis said."

"And mouths too."

The cusp: ethics of the learning curve

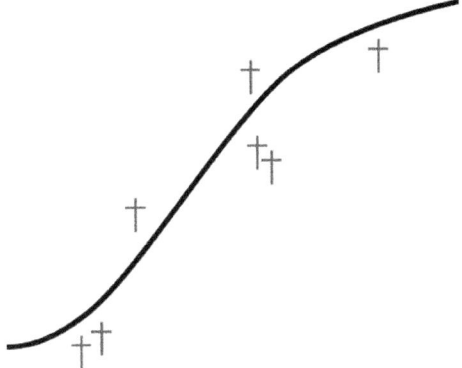

There is a moment in medical training when you think you are ready to go it alone. The difficulty is deciding when that moment has arrived. Independence, working without supervision, is a watershed moment.

Imagine this situation. A gastroenterology registrar who believes that she is ready to deal with bleeding ulcers receives a phone call. A patient is bleeding in the ER. She makes arrangements to bring the patient to the endoscopy unit. She decides not to call her consultant because he has said on a number of occasions that she is ready. He has 'signed her off'. The patient now awaits her; she takes the endoscope and passes it into his mouth. She finds the ulcer quickly and knows what to do. But it is bleeding rapidly, and the views that she obtains are not very clear. She knows what to do. She washes the ulcer, tries to clean the blood away, but still it bleeds. She begins to feel nervous…even more nervous. She asks for a needle with which to inject adrenaline, hoping that this will slow the bleeding down. Then she might see enough to apply some definitive therapy, a clip or thermal coagulation.

She waits for the endoscopy nurse to get things ready, and watches the patient. The elderly man is sedated, but his pulse rate continues to climb despite the blood transfusion. The registrar knows that she would rather her supervisor was here. But then she reflects - this is what independence is about. Coming out of your comfort zone, absorbing the stress, dealing with the situation, making the decisions, …enlarging that zone… making yourself better so you can treat the next patient with even greater confidence and skill. But what if that process involves putting this frail man at risk? She readies herself for the next part of the procedure. She knows that if this goes well she will emerge from that room a better doctor.

The scenario can now go one of two ways...

A. She injects the adrenaline and as she had hoped it has a constricting effect on the blood vessels, causing the flow to slow down. Now when she washes the blood away it takes longer to ooze back, and she can see the culprit in the middle. A raw artery that has been eroded by acid. She chooses to use the heater probe and asks the nurse to make it ready. She passes it down the channel of the endoscope until she can see it emerge on the screen. With one hand she controls the wheels on the endoscope to optimise the position, and with the other she presses the heater probe onto the vessel. Then, with her right foot she presses a pedal on the floor and sends electricity into the probe, creating a tiny zone of intense heat until the vessel is 'cooked'. Thinking that she has sealed artery she pulls the probe away. But the bleeding is even worse now. She must have torn the wall away. Quickly she calls for a clip and the nurse passes her the kit. The registrar pulls out the heater probe and quickly, calmly, replaces it with the clip delivery device. Soon she sees the metal jaws, grossly magnified, floating around the field of scarlet on the TV screen, and although the view is flooding with blood again she can still glimpse the artery. Before the window of opportunity has passed she pushes the clip onto the artery and asks the nurse to deploy. The clip closes down on the artery and stops the bleeding immediately. The field clears and she places two more clips above and below. The patient is stable.

"Well done," says the nurse "that wasn't easy. You could tackle anything now."

B. She continues to wash away the blood, but the view is terrible. She injects adrenaline and it slows things down, improving the view. Now the time is right to use the heater probe. She places its tip on the ulcer, right on the vessel that is spurting blood, and presses the pedal. The heat dissipates into the pool of blood, and makes little difference. She knows that a clip is the next best thing, but she needs a better view. She readies the clip, and through the other channel of the endoscope she squirts more water. The view improves and when the time is right she deploys the clip. For a while she thinks that the job is done, she sighs in relief and smiles at the nurse, but 30 seconds later the bleeding erupts again and all views are lost. She takes out the camera, bleeps another member of staff to come and help look after the patient, and rings a surgeon. He arrives quickly, but argues that the patient is too frail to undergo an operation. The registrar argues back, saying that she can do no more within the scope. They debate the pros and cons of various other treatments, and in the end agree that surgery is the only hope. The patient is anaesthetised and in the operating theatre 40 minutes later. The ulcer is located and sealed. But he does badly after the operation, and develops a chest infection. He remains on a ventilator, and in the end, seven days later, dies.

The registrar describes all this to her consultant. From the description he can see no reason for her to blame herself.

"You did fine." he says, "You knew when to give up, that's half the skill." He doubts that his presence would have made much of a difference. But the registrar knows that the patient's greatest chance of survival would have been afforded if he *had not had to have an operation*, if the most experienced person had been there to treat the ulcer...if she had not proceeded on her own.

*

As a trainee approaches the top of a learning curve the moment comes when they have to decide if it is safe to go it alone – the cusp. The patient who comes into hospital on that day will have no idea that they represent a significant moment in the career of the doctor who is called to perform their procedure. They will have no idea where they lie on that learning curve, or that they might form a stepping stone to independence and immaturity. This would not matter if their risk of harm was no greater than that of any other patient having the procedure. But it is the result of this risk analysis that forms a perfect example of how we balance individual risks versus societal benefits in medicine.

The concept of the learning curve was introduced to many members of the public in a horribly vivid way during the Bristol Heart scandal. One of the paediatric heart surgeons involved said,

"I believe that the reality of the learning curve may be illustrated by the evolution of surgery for transposition of the Great Arteries in this country ... in the late 80s and the very early 90s it was generally understood and accepted that when a unit introduced the Arterial Switch operation for neonates there would initially be a period of disappointing results."

I am not concerned with such extreme examples here, but the essence pertains. In order to achieve complete expertise it is necessary to accept a degree of 'trial and error'. Or is it?

*

A thorough enquiry into this subject was undertaken by a US paper, the Dallas News, following controversial reports coming out of Parkland Memorial Hospital, the primary teaching institution of University of Texas Southwestern Medical school. This hospital seemed to take a liberal attitude to the surgical training, crediting its juniors with autonomy to proceed with many operations unsupervised.

One faculty supervisor who quit in protest said the mainly poor, minority patients of Dallas County's only public hospital had effectively become "clinical fodder."

Apparently,

The head of UT Southwestern's general surgery residency program once said it was "OK for residents to make mistakes" on patients "even if they could have been avoided with better faculty supervision," according to notes taken by a faculty surgeon and later included in court records. Tim Doke, UT Southwestern's spokesman, challenged the accuracy of that account. But Anderson has testified that some faculty believed "that's how people learn," though he said he disagreed with the philosophy.

In this case (and the newspaper report makes excellent reading, as does this graphic summarising mortality), one supervisor became uncomfortable, and complained after he was called into a gall bladder operation too later, after a irreversible damage had been done to the bile duct.

This controversy crystallises an ethical dilemma in medical training. As the journalists put it, "There's good for the patient, and there's a societal good. We can't exist as a society without physicians learning on the ground."

A questionnaire study published in the BMJ found that 86% of surgical trainees or young consultants had performed procedures for the *first time* without direct supervision. This appears to be the reality of medical education. Attempts have been made to resolve the dilemma, another BMJ paper seeking to lay out a framework based on respect for the individual, beneficence and non-maleficence. In their introduction Jagsi and Lehmann explain that...

The burdens of medical education are not currently distributed fairly. In one US study, students saw disproportionately high numbers of non-white patients and patients with Medicaid (public insurance for the indigent).Another study found that children of doctor parents were less likely to be seen by trainees than were other children.

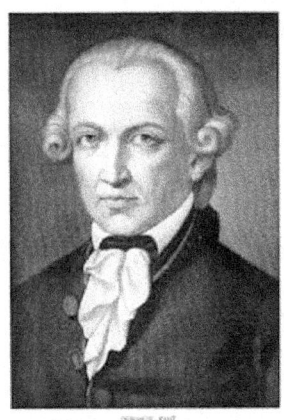

Immanuel Kant (image from Wikipedia)

However, the approach laid out in this paper does not really equip trainees with a practical method of making decisions on the spot. Another paper (Journal of Medical Ethics) approaches the problem by applying Immanuel Kant's Second Formulation of the Categorical Imperative,

"Act so that you use humanity, as much in your own person as in the person of every other, always at the same time as end and never merely as means"

In reality however,

This conflict arises because, at least presently, medical practitioners can only acquire certain skills and abilities by practising on live, human patients, and given the inevitability and ubiquity of learning curves, this learning requires some patients to be treated only as a

means to this end....Accordingly, until a way is found to reconcile them, we conclude that the Kantian ideal is inconsistent with the reality of medical practice.

To resolve this conflict,

...supervisors might undertake to delegate only under conditions where they can be as sure as possible that the procedure would be done as well as they could do it themselves. If this assurance can truly be given by the supervising doctor, then the conflict is solved.'

This seems unrealistic. So are the patients who take their place on our learning curves nothing more than a means to an end? The paper begins with a quotation from Atul Gawande's book <u>Complications: a surgeon's notes on an imperfect science</u>

'To fail to adopt new techniques would mean denying patients meaningful medical advances. Yet the perils of the learning curve are inescapable—no less in practice than in residency'

Le Morvan and Stock seek to challenge the perception that patients are guinae pigs in four ways;

1) **Discontinuing unnecessary use of patients without consent** - they suggest that we introduce a consent process where possible. The example of pelvic examinations by students on anaesthetised patients is one such example.

2) Continuing to develop **medical simulation** models

3) **Enhancing supervision**, but..."We are sceptical that such an approach, applied stringently, is practical for all procedures. It is hard to imagine—for example, that an experienced surgeon can honestly say that his trainee's first liver biopsy will be performed just as well as he would perform it himself. Moving in this direction, toward a more conservative educational model, would, however, reduce the extent to which patients are used as means only."

4) **Changing expectations, or universalising** the problem. If the involvement of trainees is taken into account when the statistical outcome from a procedure is calculated, patients waiting for that procedure are not actually being disadvantaged by having performed by a trainee. This argument does have a whiff of sophistry about it, but I have found myself using

it before. As a patient and a parent I would want the hospital's best qualified person to treat me or my children (although I am probably too polite to demand as much), but as a trainee I often muttered to myself, in response to a patient's underwhelmed expression, "Look, either I do this procedure or it's another five hour wait...what will it be?" As the authors conclude,

It does, however, offer a useful way of approximating this ideal in light of the constraints imposed by the reality of medical practice.

I don't think there is a way of truly resolving the Kantian conflict unless our patients accept that it is not possible to always see the most qualified person in the institution. But the deal must be reciprocated by trainees – they must ensure that every single clinical interaction is approached not from the point of view of 'polishing their resume' (as the Dallas News article put it), but from the point of view of the patient. The trainee may well be on the cusp, there may be a theoretically increased risk, but if the skills are embedded, if the trainers have given their blessing, if they feel ready on that particular day or night…no more can be asked.

Blaming patients: a very human temptation

Being human, doctors sometimes blame others when things go wrong. Because they spend most of their time interacting with patients, there is a temptation to blame them. The purist might argue that a patient can *never* be responsible for suboptimal care, medical error or lifestyle associated disease, but the issue is complicated and deserving of examination. The word blame not only implies *fault*, indicating that harm is directly related to a person's actions or omissions, but that they are not deserving of sympathy. If we accept that sympathy is a necessary precursor to empathy, through the stirring of compassion and the will to do the emotional work that is required, its absence could compound a patient's sense of isolation and vulnerability. Responsibility is a more subtle term, but its effect is the same – the shifting expectation away from the doctor and towards the patient. But patients *do* have to take some responsibility for their condition and their care. Where does the balance lie?

In this article I will explore various situations in which doctors might find themselves blaming patients. These move from the immediacy of the clinical interface to societal attitudes to lifestyle and 'deservingness'.

1. Passivity or fear?

Imagine this scenario. A 34 year old man, working, busy, sees a specialist complaining of weight loss and night sweats. A CT scan is organised, and the patient waits for the follow up appointment. It never comes. He waits, and waits... losing weight, feeling ill. Six weeks later he goes back to his GP who makes contact with the specialist, leaving a message with his secretary. Three days later the patient is called at home by the secretary who offers him an appointment *next day*. The young patient attends, and is informed that the scan shows large volume lymphadenopathy which must represent lymphoma. He needs an urgent excision biopsy and chemotherapy. The tumour is extensive, and six weeks more advanced than it needed to be before commencing treatment. The patient asks what happened. The specialist apologises profusely - the system usually flags up abnormal scans, he can't explain why this one slipped through. But sitting there, looking at the pale, thin young man, the specialist thinks to himself,

'But why, for heaven's sake, didn't you chase it up?'

Was the patient remiss here? Yes, the system let him down, but would he have left it six weeks before getting back in touch with the manufacturer of a new television after it had been reported as faulty. Why not call the hospital? Why not call the consultant's office and make a fuss?

Or consider this: a 54 year old female with cirrhosis and ascites (fluid collecting in the abdomen) is prescribed strong diuretics or water tablets. Three weeks after starting the treatment she comes to the clinic for a review and routine blood tests to ensure that her kidneys are not being 'squeezed'. She looks unwell to the consultant, nauseated, her eye sockets sunken. There is not an ounce of excess fluid on her body. The consultant hands her a request form and emphasises that is *vital* that she go straight to the phlebotomy room for her blood test, and that he will contact her the next day to advise on the dose of diuretics. He explains that he may even need to stop them if the kidneys are being damaged. She has the blood tests. That night the consultant, who happens to be on call, is called in to an emergency. It takes all night to sort out, and he works through the day until it is time to go home. It is Friday evening. Suddenly, on Sunday morning, he remembers the blood test. He calls the hospital and gets the house office on duty to check the results system.

'Funny,' says the junior doctor, 'It says she's actually an in-patient.'

'What ward?'

'Intensive care...'

The consultant calls ICU. His patient was admitted that morning, in advanced renal failure. She is now on dialysis - hopefully a temporary measure. As he breaks the connection the consultant scrolls through the reminders and alerts on his mobile phone; yes, there it is, reminding him to check those results at midday on the Friday. Why didn't he hear it? Who knows? His system, his fail-safe…failed. He sits down, at home, curses himself, but reflects – 'Why the hell didn't the lab call me on Friday...and why didn't *she* call my office...I told her those results were vital, they were needed to change her dose...but she waited, and waited, getting sicker and sicker...'

Was she to blame? Wouldn't it be reasonable to have expected her to be interested, curious, worried? The consultant said he would get back to her, but he didn't. Wasn't that a sign that he had forgotten? And if he had forgotten, wouldn't it have been prudent to remind him? Why the passivity?

The question of passivity opens up a deep box of psychology and potential explanations - the traditions of paternalism which engender an unquestioning acceptance of how the system reviews and communicates results; fear of the monolith, of how the hospital will react to prods and questions; denial, that anything is wrong; superstition, in that actively *asking* for results will actually alter one's chances of receiving bad news. These are aspects of a patient's psychology, and are responses to illness. It may not be reasonable to expect patients to take as much responsibility for their own bodies than they would for something (such as the new television) that cannot threaten their physical wellbeing. Rational thought, logical responses and proactive behaviour may be blunted by the normal response to illness.

2. Blaming the body if not the person

Writing on the KevinMD website a patient by the name of Warmsocks described how she had been 'blamed' for being too sensitive to a painkilling drug, Tramadol. In fact she had not been advised on how to titrate the dose correctly, but this example reminded me of a reaction I have witnessed in other doctors, and have been guilty of myself. That of instantly shifting the blame for an unexpected complication or reaction to an aspect of the patient's physiology or anatomy. That is not to say the patient is blamed *personally*. Examples might include 'anomalous anatomy', an allergy that had not been previously 'declared', or a co-existing condition that had not been revealed during the initial history. The patient is not held responsible, but nor is the doctor. Data was missing, no-one is to blame...not you...and definitely not me!

An example: patients' responses to intravenous sedation vary widely. If a patient remains inadequately sedated despite receiving the maximum permitted dose, their experience of a procedure may be unpleasant and psychologically harmful. In the field of endoscopy this is a commonly encountered situation. After the procedure an explanation might sound like this –

'I hope that wasn't too bad. You didn't seem very sleepy.'

'I felt everything. I heard everything.'

'I'm sorry. But I gave as much as I could.'

'Why didn't it work?'

'Well, people react differently. We don't know why. Peoples' metabolism varies, their sensitivity to drugs…'

'So it was me. A low pain threshold?'

'No, it was nothing you could influence…'

The doctor's explanation is partially defensive, for he does not feel entirely culpable for his patient's poor experience. But in referring to the patient's metabolism he has handed the 'blame' right back into the patient's lap, to do with it what she will. However impersonal the a word like 'metabolism', the patient will go home feeling that the nature of her reaction was down to *her*. Although the doctor thought that he was being non-pejorative, the take home message may have been entirely personal.

3. Justification after unexpected death

When a patient dies unexpectedly, despite the best efforts of the team, a sense of failure ensues. There is regret, there is sadness, there is self-examination. While reflecting on what went wrong and what might have been done better it is not uncommon for a distancing to occur. This is especially common if members of the team express guilt. A discussion might sound something like this -

'How are you feeling?' asks a consultant of her house officer, a day after a middle aged patient dies.

'I don't understand why it happened. We diagnosed his infection promptly, gave the right treatment, escalated to intensive care...what did we do wrong?'

'We didn't do anything wrong. You didn't do anything wrong. I'd tell you if there was something that could have been done differently.'

'So why did *he* die while the patient we had with an identical infection, three weeks ago, survived? And that patient was much older.'

'There are reasons behind the way patients respond to illness that we don't fully understand. Some people develop overwhelming sepsis, some just get a mild fever.'

'So it was something unique to him?'

'I don't know. All I know is we gave the same treatment to those two patients and one died and one survived. It wasn't down to us. So don't blame yourself...'

So who should she blame? No-one. It's not a question of *fault*. But in looking for reasons, for justification, it is natural to seek a focus for the negative reaction that death, failure, causes. This is blame. In the discussion presented here that blame is directed back to the deceased patient, for the idiosyncratic way in which his body responded to the infection. Not a strong form of blame, but a definite transference of responsibility.

4. A step to the right

An internet tour of medical blame will take you down the road of 'self-inflicted' disease. That is the group of conditions that can be attributed to lifestyle, choices and an unwillingness to change behaviour.

[Dr Peter Attia gave an emotional TED talk](#) on the epiphany that occurred when he developed features of the metabolic syndrome, causing a painful juxtaposition with the lack of empathy, perhaps even a degree of contempt, he had experienced when treating obese patients. He blamed them, and felt less sympathy for them than he did for other apparently more deserving patients. However, not all clinicians will go through such a conversion, and policy makers working at a remove from such patients have begun to build blame into the health care system.

In the US, as described in a blog post by Bob Doherty recently ('Stop blaming patients for not doing enough to stay healthy') a philosophy of blame can be manifested by increased health insurance for some groups, or rather sinister sounding 'health contingent wellness programmes' which have been objected to by House Democrats. As Bob Doherty says,

'…many of these things – eating better, exercising more, not smoking, not drinking to excess–may be very difficult or even impossible for some people to achieve because of genetics (family history of alcoholism and other substance abuse), culture and community (the diet your grew up with, the food choices available to you in your community, exposure to crime and violence), stress, literacy, physical and emotional abuse, how you were raised by your parents, the quality of your schools–the list goes on and on.'

In the UK the most vivid example of converting blame to policy comes from Conservative MP and part-time GP Dr Phillip Lee, who in 2012 hit the headlines by suggesting that patients with type 2 diabetes may need to pay for prescriptions – "If you want to have doughnuts for breakfast, fine,' he said,' but there is a cost implication down the line,". The operative word is 'want'. Do patients *want* to eat rich food, or smoke, or drink? Yes. Do they *want* to be obese, get lung cancer or die of cirrhosis? No. There may be a mechanistic line between the lifestyle habit and the disease, but breaking it requires more than admonition or financial penalty. Blame when applied to addiction, be it to food, alcohol or drugs, is a dangerous word.

5. Can blame exist without freedom?

Lifestyles driven by addiction and compulsion take us into the area of 'moral responsibility'. A paper by Rebecca Brown called 'Moral responsibility for (un) healthy behaviour' identifies -

'…a growing trend for 'responsibilisation' (often related to 'personalised healthcare') which assumes that agents can (and should) be held morally responsible for their health outcome

but then challenges 'one key assumption...that, in determining their own lifestyles, individuals act freely and are morally responsible for engaging in unhealthy behaviours' and seeks to 'question the legitimacy of holding agents morally responsible for their (un)healthy lifestyles.'

She describes an approach in which

credit be awarded according to the extent to which agents 'conscientiously strive' to do the right thing.

while acknowledging,

that an agent's capacity to 'strive' may be influenced by her upbringing and social circumstances: factors out of her control and not her responsibility.

This reminds me of my own practise in liver medicine. The clearest instance of blame is seen in the arena of alcohol addiction. It is common for a patient to survive a life threatening episode of alcohol induced liver failure, and on discharge the doctor will say,

'That was very close. If you drink again, even a glass, you will probably die.'

The patient comes back into hospital 6 weeks later, in liver failure. His partner admits that he has been drinking heavily. How much clearer can it be – the patient is to blame, surely! Then comes the question of whether the patient should be offered the chance of organ support on the intensive care unit. Their 'deservingness' *may* be taken into account. The impression of deservingness might rely on the efforts that they have made to give up alcohol. Are they in a programme? Did they take the seriousness of their last scrape with death to heart and throw away the bottles when they got home. Is this the tenth such admission? In asking ourselves these questions we are therefore tempted into ascribing to ourselves the roles of moral judge and jury. But we must be aware that the General Medical Council, in Good Medical Practice, says,

"The investigations or treatment you provide or arrange must be based on the assessment you and the patient make of their needs and priorities, and on your clinical judgement about the likely effectiveness of the treatment options. You must not refuse or delay treatment because you believe that a patient's actions have contributed to their condition..."

With this in mind, is it ever defensible to cite a patient's pattern of behaviour, his intractable addiction or compulsion, in denying a particular form of treatment? No. But if that behaviour is felt to make the chance of a successful outcome less likely, or minimal, then it *becomes* acceptable to deny treatment. If ongoing alcoholism will inevitably lead to recurrent disease, or continued smoking will fur up the newly fashioned coronary vessels...these may well strong enough reasons to justify that harsh calculation.

Rebecca Brown goes on to explore how much behaviour is 'habitual' and unconscious, such that 'A large and sustained psychological effort is needed to intervene in everyday behaviours and alter habits.' And the success of such efforts may depend on social factor, there being evidence to show that – 'smokers from the most deprived socioeconomic groups are as likely to attempt to quit smoking (and to seek help in doing so), but are only half as likely to succeed compared with those in the highest socioeconomic groups'.

Lastly she explores the concept of 'freedom' to choose, referring to the philosopher and political theorist Philip Pettit's work 'A Theory of Freedom: from psychology to the politics of agency' he suggests a person is fit to be held responsible for their behaviour if:

- their actions are genuinely free rather than forced (by compulsion)
- they can identify with the things that they do (for example, a patient may 'find themselves' smoking despite making great efforts to give up, almost as though it is another person doing it) and,
- their actions are theirs and not an action produced under pressure from others – the availability and the prominence of high calorie fast foods in deprived environments where cravings for such foods might be higher, could be interpreted as an example.

6. I am innocent

A study by Alison Chapple and colleagues, 'Stigma, shame, and blame experienced by patients with lung cancer: qualitative study' provides insights into how the perception of blame can affect patients. Sometimes we can get it wrong, and the patient was in fact 'innocent', as here -

When I went to see an oncologist for further treatments because I'd had an operation and I'd had half of my left lung removed, I asked them what he thought had caused it and he just laughed and said, "That's obvious, through smoking." And my wife who was with me at the time, and we've been together since we were 14, she just said, "Well he's never smoked." So right away what annoyed me as well as that, on my medical records I'm classed as a smoker and every time I ever went for review after that they would ask me, "Are you still smoking?" because that's down there. And no matter how I told them, I'd say, "Look I don't want that on there, I never smoked."

Casting blame, whether overtly by verbally attributing disease to prior actions, or covertly by just thinking that the patient is at fault, is a dangerous game. You might be completely wrong. What is more, even if you are assured that the patient *has* contributed to their own illness, you have no idea what lies at the source of their behaviour. The question needs to be asked - would you have successfully avoided addiction to alcohol, nicotine or calories if you had grown up in the same environment, with the same pressures, temptations and opportunities? Would you regard yourself as 'innocent'?

Conclusion

I have tried to show that it is natural for doctors to apportion blame. Even if we conclude that it is not justified we must accept that it *will* happen. I write this a doctor who as experienced all of the emotional reactions described above - I am not immune!

The dangers of giving in to the temptation of blame in the clinical setting are those of alienating patients, undermining empathy and disrupting the therapeutic relationship. In the wider social or political context the dangers are stigmatisation and the risk of unjust health policies. It seems that this natural, and therefore inescapable response to illness represents an ever-present threat to optimum medical practice. The solution? This must be down to a combination of professionalism, whereby doctors compartmentalise their emotional reactions and the way they behave, and advocacy. But that is not enough. Being a good doctor requires *positive* emotional work, understanding, liking, sympathising, commiserating and finding, together with the patient, the best route through a difficult situation. Merely tolerating a patient whom one blames for their predicament is not enough. Any sense of blame needs to be *suppressed* and dissociated entirely from the doctor's approach to the relationship. Fate has thrown them in your path, as a professional, and if you will not do your utmost to understand them and help them, who will?

NHS1

NHS2 on the year 2053: a sideways look at the future

The Hub headquarters, glass clad and monolithic, glistened from its dominant position at the north end of the campus. I stared up at it, but was soon drawn back to the shabby, warehouse-like building to my right which appeared to have received little attention since the winter of '45, the year I had worked in it as an intensive care doctor. We called it the 'Lung' back then.

A new influenza strain had swept through the country, the largest epidemic since 1918/19, and most of those infected developed respiratory failure. Because there was a national shortage of ventilators we relied on five powerful, central bellows [A] to pump oxygen via filtered tubes into fifty intubated patients at a time. It was hell. Two trainee doctors and eight nurses looked after each fifty patient cohort. It was one of the reasons I packed it all in. Each morning as I walked in, and each night as I walked back to the magnatram terminal, I saw the lighted windows of the *other* unit, where patients slept, artificially, to the sound of *their own* machine.

Six months later I gave up medicine to become a social historian. And that's why I had returned, to the North Eastern Health Hub - to conduct research for my new book. The Hub had grown while its competitors in the region had closed down…or, more accurately, had been absorbed. The medical staff moved across, local managers evaporated, the bricks and mortar were flattened. The magnatram was jammed with patients arriving for their appointments. The Hub was massive now - a hospital town.

As the lift approached the executive floor I began to get nervous. Professor Sam Laszlo, or his PA, had put aside forty-five minutes. In that time I had to discover all I could about how his company had come to dominate the UK health market. I knew he would be coy about some things…but I hoped that pride would feed his honesty.

He smiled openly, his tall silhouette framed and blurred in window of bright blue sky behind him.

"Hello! Thank you for coming today. I'm sorry we don't have much time…"

"Any insights would be gratefully received…it's a bit of a coup to get to meet you."

" I understand you worked here once."

"Yes. Intensive care. In the Lung."

"The Lung?"

"Down there." I pointed over his shoulder, for the roof was visible below us.

"Ah. Of course. I apologise. It's got a quite different use now."

"It looks pretty neglected to me."

"Not on the inside. Not at all. It houses the fibreoptic data spine, and the refrigeration units to keep the hardware cool. Since the UniRec[B] scandal we have had to keep all patient data on-site. A pain, but there you go. Anyway, tell me, remind me, what is title of your book? You sent it to me but I don't have it with me."

"'Two Tears: The Long Dying of NHS1'. But I might change it. That's 'tears' with an E and an A."

"Two Tears! Ingenious! But why not 'In Pursuit Of Excellence: How NHS2 Put The Patient Back In Charge?"

"I err…come from a rather socialist background. I'm cynical about the changes…"

"But it was New Labour who let us in. You won't remember personally of course, but after Cameron won a large majority for the Old Conservatives in '15, on a welfare-immigration ticket, ably assisted by the nascent economic recovery, New Labour begged David Miliband to come back from the States. He shook them up, rode the economic recovery and promised a happier life free of austerity…and they won in 2020. Small majority mind you. The new health secretary, Burnham, was held by a few to the promise he had made in 2012 to repeal the Health and Social Care Act, but it was too late [1]. The benefits had become clear. It was the quality you see. New Labour didn't even have to discuss health in their manifesto, there was no hunger for change anymore. People were happy."

"The healthy majority were happy."

"No, patients were happy. Qualified Providers came in, staffed their establishments properly, asked their patients about the experience, changed what they didn't like, dealt with complaints promptly, sacked doctors and nurses in the lowest 5% on their real-time bedside compassion scores...how could Burnham dismantle it? Private companies were soon providing 25% of secondary care, it was growing at several percentage points per year. Trusts all over the country had budgeted for huge increases in income from privately ensured patients [2]. It was done."

"But by that time there was evidence of inaccessibility..."

"*No-one* was excluded. Remember, the state was still funding healthcare – and increasing it - as it does now, no-one *had* to pay anything to get treatment..."

"Isn't that disingenuous? State funding fell in proportion to national health needs estimates, provision became second class. This was described in the Scott review in 2024. There were already identifiable, statistically significant survival differences between NHS and privately insured patients..."

"In a few conditions only."

"Cancer..."

"But cancer is no longer an issue, not in the era of vectorgen therapy. By 2022 that technology was already coming through. Successive governments saw that and planned strategically to account for a reduction in demand. A poor example...for your book. Don't hang your thesis on cancer. The story isn't in mortality, it's in quality of life. Private companies were soon demonstrating a greater focus of quality of life..."

"...because those companies concentrated on the non life-threatening conditions. The routine, relatively safe stuff...non-urgent surgery for healthy people. That's how you get great Patient Reported Outcome Measures."

"How can you say that? What are we most famous for?"

"Hegemony."

"We are dominant now, I agree. But clinically?"

"The HEPMatrix, I guess."

"Yes! We poured resources into a group of patients with high mortality, very little hope, that no-one had tried to help before, and we changed the game. What happens now when alcoholics or Hepatitis Q^C patients decompensate? They are plugged into the HEPMatrix until they recover. It's revolutionised the care of liver failure. My predecessor in this office was awarded the Nobel prize. I won't accept this overwhelming negativity. We do benefit society…we make money yes, but we re-invest…"

"You have to re-invest, to create new markets. The HEPMatrix did that. It opened up a massive market, and the state had no choice but to pay you to provide the machines."

"The HEPMatrix would never have come about without private investment. You must understand that. We ran research programmes from the outset. It's altruistic, clearly."

"Are drug companies truly altruistic? No. It's their business. Health is your business. You wouldn't invest in research unless, on balance, you made money out of it."

"The two are intertwined. Healthcare has never come for free, somebody pays. Just as we pay for food, water, energy, CO_2 removal…you grew up regarding clean air and a stable climate as basic human rights, but twenty-five years ago, when you were what – three or four years old? - we were all taxed for those electrolised graphene spongestacks you see on the horizon. Every industrialised country in the world did the same after the Mumbai Olympics were washed out and the European drought of 2026/27. Health does not come for free. Someone must make money out of it, but as long as that money is made ethically, and used well, what's the problem? My shareholders are not evil men and women. They work. They too will get sick someday."

"And none of them will go state."

"It's so lacking in objectivity, your line of questioning…"

"I have a responsibility to dig. In the time we have I've got to stress my sources a little bit…do you mind? I want to know about the separation. What precipitated the overt separation of state and private funded health streams? It's not something you find written about much."

"It's convoluted. When the double-prion phenomenon began to reveal itself in the huge wave of pre-senile dementia, it became clear that disease progression could be halted if the diagnosis could be made within six months of disease onset and a course of three, 72 hour extra-corporeal cerebrospinal fluid fractionations. General practitioners were urged to screen their patients, and this led to a massive increase in referrals to neurology clinics around the country…"

"…and the true two-speed nature of New Health Streaming (NHS2) was revealed."

"Quite. It had been going on for years of course, that's what the Streaming structure was all about…but the double-prion epidemic, Marshall's disease[D], showed up its...vulnerabilities."

"You mean only those who were insured got seen and treated in time."

"Only a condition with such a short window of therapeutic opportunity could have done it."

"How thoughtless of it."

"It could not have been planned for."

"But it happened. New diseases occur all the time. Whatever system we have needs to be able to handle them, equitably."

"NHS2 was doing just that, both streams were audited and proven to work within clinically acceptable timescales. Until then there were no real inequalities…"

"…until the McCartney report smashed that illusion. She showed, five years later, that among the uninsured permanent dementia was eight times as prevalent than among the insured. Because they didn't get seen in time. Two streams…"

"New Health Streaming was developed democratically, in the oldest parliament in the world. The populace agreed, in principle, that those in work, and therefore insured, should be seen sooner, as their health was more important to the community. You think that's evil…the voting public did not. How else do you think the Cameron government, the government that facilitated and welcomed the arrival of Any Qualified Providers, how else do you think they got voted in again in 2015? They had a mandate by then, and New Labour *did not* reverse it."

"I don't believe the populace always reach the right decision."

"Ahh! So perhaps a Communist regime, ruled by wise oligarchs who know what is best for their people, would suit you better! That went well in the mid 20th!"

It was going a bit wrong by now. I glanced at my watch and saw that time was running out. The professor looked down at the glass surface of his desk. I watched his eye track a new message, but I could not read the words from where I sat.

"How interesting!" he exclaimed, looking up sharply, "I know more about than you realise. You *do* have an agenda after all. Care to tell me about it, or shall I tell you what I know?"

"What do you know?"

"Your mother succumbed to complications following the removal of her colon…an operation she asked to have after receiving the result of a LifeSpan assessment. You've been politically active since your late teens. Demonstrations, i-pamphlets…and then you worked here. In the 'Lung'. If I had known all that I wouldn't have…"

"Seen me?"

"I don't know. How old were you when she died?"

"Seven."

"That was what, early 30's, we had just published the Picasso[E] paper. A little earlier and perhaps she wouldn't have given Lifespan as much credence."

"Well she did. It gave her an 89% lifetime bowel cancer risk, with a high chance it would be biologically aggressive and unamenable to early detection, curative surgery or vectorgen therapy. It's understandable, what she did."

"Our analysis of Picasso's DNA gave him a 79% chance of a similar disease. And he lived to a good age. Tragic."

"But your company owned LifeSpan."

"We sold it after the first cohort of adverse prophylactic procedures."

"Five years later. After thousands of unnecessary procedures."

"Not all were unnecessary. Many people were saved. That's a fact. Once again, your Manichean view is proved to be naïve. It's all about balance. Society, which includes this company, wavers across the correct path, to the left and to the right, as it develops new technologies and discovers how to apply them, but the correct path can only be charted in retrospect. Don't blame the innovators."

Click

The tape recorder in my jacket pocket had run out.

"Tape! How quaint. Of course, your G-glasses would have been taken off you downstairs. The screener would never detect a *tape recorder*. But you should have just asked, the audio file would have been in your cloud before you opened the door to leave. It still can be. I'm not embarrassed."

"Is that it then?"

"I think so. Don't you? I hope it been useful."

Footnotes

A – The bellows were steeped in irony. The Hub had brought them in a few years before the influenza epidemic hit to manage the Guillaine-Barre outbreak of '42, itself caused by a faulty influenza vaccine. The chief executive in charge of the manufacturing company who signed off the use of cheap porcine substrates (leading to xenomyelinic cross-talk) is still in punitive re-profiling on the North Sea hulk-network.

B - The ill-fated attempt to provide a unified system with which to access the medical records of all patients, nationwide, had a promising start. UniRec rolled out in 2024 and received positive reviews from primary and secondary care. Patients too were able to access their medical details from home and on their smart devices. However the financial regulator, while investigating the stellar performance of a private insurance provider, Longevity+, in the financial year 2027/8 discovered that the confidential medical details of over 80% of their applicants had been accessed. All those rejected for insurance cover had early indicators, in their bio-informatics, of chronic disease susceptibility. After this scandal UniRec was dismantled and all physical and wireless connections between regional databanks were severed or firewalled.

C- Hepatitis Q was discovered in 2038. It was identified, retrospectively, in archived biological material as far back as 1987. Although blood borne, the virus did not appear to have been passed to blood transfusion recipients, probably due to its exquisite sensitivity to citrate, an additive used in packed red cell storage. In any case, since 2032 red cells have not been used for transfusion, the advent of Self-Terminating Oxygen Delivery Nanobots (STODNs) having made this practise obsolete. The Hep Q epidemic of the late 30's and early 40's was caused by a single infected narcotics developer who isolated and then mass produced a novel hallucinogen from his own bile.

D - The currently accepted explanation is that a new, equine prion (proper nomenclature $PrP^{eq/valupak/2012}$) was acquired through contamination of processed meat and ready-made meals in 2012/3 (and probably for several years prior to this). This interacted with the highly prevalent but latent 'new variant Creutzfeldt-Jakob' (nvCJD) prion. nvCJD was related to Bovine Spongiform Encephalopathy (BSE) which entered the human food chain in the final decade of the 20th century. Cows, natural herbivores, had been fed meat and bone meal derived from sheep infected with Scrapie, and calves which received protein supplements to accelerate growth.

E - Picasso's DNA was extracted from a bone fragment, retrieved with the permission of his estate from his grave in Vauvenargues, Eurorealm Subzone 26 (formerly Provence-Alpes-Côte d'Azur, France). LifeSpan were criticised not only for driving people to unnecessary surgery on healthy organs, but for a number of suicides (2,347, proven association) that occurred in the weeks prior to a 'likely date of death (natural causes only)' that was provided, at extra charge and without guarantee, to their clients.

References

[1] Speech to Royal College of Midwives's annual conference in Brighton, 16th November 2011

http://www.guardian.co.uk/society/2011/nov/17/labour-repeal-nhs-bill

[2] Freedom of Information requests in 2013 revealed that Trust (NHS1 terminology) planned to increase income from private patients by up to 200% or more in the first years following the Health and Social Care Act/Any Qualified Provider agreement.

http://www.guardian.co.uk/society/2013/apr/06/nhs-hospitals-increase-private-patients

Apologies and acknowledgments: Isaac Asimov, Philip K Dick, David Mitchell, Arthur C Clarke, and all serious health commentators out there.

Precious: a legacy of understaffing in healthcare

I've been catching up on Professor Don Berwick, author of the recent NHS safety review. A powerful character, with a powerful, patient centred, emotional approach to healthcare - so emotional in fact that his audiences have shed tears, and readers have cried over his essays. He has said, of the patient-physician dynamic,

"Some say doctors and patients should now be partners in care…not so, I think. In my view, we doctors are not our patients' partners; we are guests in our patients' lives."

The dinosaur in me finds it difficult to swallow that quote whole, and although I see the validity of the aspiration I know that it does not approximate to the truth for many doctors. In an (unsuccessful) consultant interview I was asked, 'Who is the most important part of the team?' I paused, thought to myself - *ah, I know what you're getting at!* - and said, 'Well, the patient.' The questioner marked his paper and nodded; right answer…move on. Did he really believe the answer? Did I really believe my answer? Did he believe that I believed my answer - or was it all political correctness? My cool reaction to Don Berwick's quote above set me thinking about the reasons why, for some, the doctor rather than the patient remains at the centre of the 'team'. In this post I will explore the theory that perennial time pressure or overwork, a manifestation of understaffing, shifts the emphasis from one of duty (to the patient, to compassionate care, to perfectionism) to one of exaggerated self-importance on the part of the doctor. If humility is a necessary foundation to compassion, and pride can contribute to medical error, there may be something in it. It's a subtle psychological trail - bear with me!

My time is precious and you're lucky to have it

As an SHO I accompanied a consultant on a post-take ward round. He approached a young man who had been admitted as an emergency overnight. The patient was talking on his mobile phone. As my consultant neared the bedside the patient looked up, nodded and carried on talking. The consultant lingered for another 10 seconds, watched as the conversation continued, and turned away, saying, "That was it his chance to see me, and he's lost it." The whole team moved on, the patient had no idea what had happened, and he never benefited a consultant level review. I sympathised with my consultant at the time. Now, looking back, I think - hang on, you are only here because patients like him come into hospital. A consultant rejecting patients because they do not show due deference is like a shopkeeper throwing out customers - you are cutting off your own livelihood.

A more quotidien example? A Foundation Year doctor wakes a patient at 3 AM to take blood for a non-urgent but overdue drug level from a patient with difficult veins. The patient complains, verbally or non-verbally, and the nurse requests that the test be deferred to the morning. The FY says, "Look, I was asked to do this when I came on duty at 9 PM, this is the first opportunity I've had, *this* is my window of opportunity…" Once again, the emphasis is on the doctor's convenience, on access to his expertise, and the patient must submit to his conditions if he wants to receive appropriate care. It's not the doctor's fault – he was seeing more urgent cases – but the system is personified in the doctor's uncompromising expression.

This sentiment carries over into the outpatient setting. A patient rearranges his day to attend a 3.45 PM appointment only to find that the clinic is running 60 minutes late. He is upset. Behind the door the doctor feels harried and rushed. She has lost control of this one, not through indolence, perhaps because three patients in a row had problems that required more than their allotted 10 or 15 minutes. When the doctor and the delayed patient meet at last, both have a grievance. The patient dare not express his (at least not to the doctor herself) for his wellbeing depends on her inclination to do the best for him, to take the utmost trouble. The pressure of time warps a relationship that is already highly skewed in terms of power and vulnerability.

'Her time is evidently precious, I'd better not ask that third question I was thinking about…I'm lucky to get any time at all by the look of this clinic…'

And for the doctor, what does the fact that this patient's autonomy has been limited, compressed by the minute hand, mean? It means the patient is dealt with in 7 minutes…because,

'…he didn't have a serious disease, he didn't <u>need</u> a twenty minute chat, and that's OK, because, damn it, my time <u>is</u> precious.'

The overrun begins to correct itself, the sky begins to clear, all is well with the world once again. That is, from the doctor's point of view.

The safety connection – 'It will have to do'

The obvious link to make between time pressure and safety is that when tasks are performed in a rush, or in a state of fatigue or distraction, important steps can be missed or bodged. I think it's more subtle than that. When doctors embark on practical procedures or a complicated analyses they are usually pretty focussed. But if that task is one of many that require completion in a set timeframe, and if the doctor's presence has been eagerly awaited by the patient or ward nurses, I wonder if that sentiment - *'You're lucky to have me, I'm needed in another five places right now!'* - can foster a tendency to be satisfied with imperfect process, technique or outcome. No one can find a sterile gown…a nurse asks for 5 minutes to pick one up from theatres; the second drug chart is off the ward – can you wait a few minutes while someone fetches it? – *'No, I'm in a hurry, I need to be somewhere else, it'll have to do!'* ***It will have to do***…the attitude that encourages compromise, the 'normalisation of deviance', the acceptance that harm is not only inevitable (which it is), but hardly worth trying to minimise.

The habit of self regard

In the days of 36 hour weekday shifts and 56 hour weekend shifts (9 AM Saturday to 5 or 6 PM Monday, no protected rest - the last time I did that was in 2002/3), the fatigue, clumsiness and emotional lability that built up during successive days and nights encouraged an inwardness, a continuous process of self-analysis and self-regard that made me the centre of each patient-doctor interaction. Sometimes this was appropriate, for example when preparing to insert a central line after 40 hours with just a few snatched moments of sleep on the sofa or the mess snooker table – it was a kind of risk assessment, *am I up to this?* But that habit, of wondering about how *I* was, how tired *I* was, how pressurised *I* was, has been a hard one to shake. It might have infected generations of doctors who now work in more relaxed circumstances, but who still approach their working day with an attitude of *'This is how much I've got to give, I'm the important one here, take it or leave it.'*

Service Starts Here

I was once told that in a United States hospital the staff wore name badges with little flaps which, when lifted, revealed the words *'Service Starts Here'* printed underneath. When I heard this I laughed. It just didn't make sense. Service? You call what we do in the middle of the night a service? We're not hotel concierges, we're doctors! But now, having read so much about how patients have suffered indignities or harms in NHS hospitals, I think I can see how a diminished sense of service can lead to a diminished sense of respect, for patients. The arguments above might go some way to explaining that. But it has to be recognised that lack of any resource leads to a seller's market, where those have the expertise or skill that appears to be in such high demand can adopt whatever attitude they like. The patients will always come, they have no real choice in an emergency.

During my career I have witnessed huge improvements in junior doctors' working hours, and I am hopeful that these will allow the sense of duty or service to thrive in future generations. I fear that for many doctors, whose formative years predated these reforms, the psychological consequences of being forever behind, forever tired, forever in demand, forever desperately *needed*, will continue to cast patients in the role of supplicants. In order to break down that sentient, and assimilate Berwick's comment about being mere guests, it is necessary to downplay that sense of significance. As we pass through the lives of others, we need to tread carefully and take great care. They have not come to the hospital to see *us*, but to get better, and we just happen to be the ones they meet when they get there.

Journeymen: why aren't doctors more loyal to the NHS?

The NHS is being dismantled, privatised, on that I think most are agreed. There appears to be a groundswell of resistance to this, at least there does if you spend time on Twitter. Here socially engaged, predominantly left wing commentators rally to the cause, but beyond the Twittersphere the story does not seem to attract much attention. The BBC is not interested, the press explore it fitfully. Anger is contained. It looks like a done deal. But what of those who work for the NHS? Surely doctors and nurses are fighting, demonstrating, complaining. I don't see them. Do they have no loyalty? I'm not out there either. Do I?

The Luminous Bed Test

One way of assessing a person's attitude to the NHS is to ask, in the manner of a market researcher, how they *felt* during the Olympic opening ceremony. You would assume that most health care professionals felt proud when those illuminated beds lined up to spell out the letters 'N H S' for the whole world to see. For me it was an abstract kind of pride. Perhaps that was because the Health and Social Care Act had already received royal assent, and many had identified it as the beginning of the end. Danny Boyle's choreography seemed like a cheeky, even subversive attempt to signify national affection for a lost cause. The impression was not helped by the news (released before the Olympics were even over) that Trusts were being encouraged to export 'the NHS brand'. It was that superficial term that caused me to ask myself - *What does the NHS mean to me?* To answer that requires an examination of my relationship with the NHS. And, like most employee-employer relationships, it's complicated.

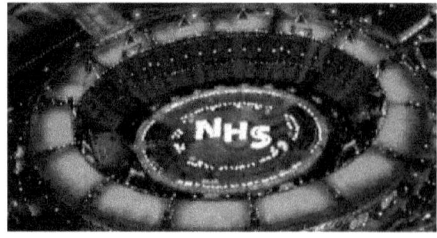

Aerial view of Olympic opening ceremony

Mixed feelings

Doctors, especially those in training, have not always been treated well by the NHS. Until recently the hours were hellish. Now the hours are better but the team-working ethos has been fragmented. Trainees struggle to find the time to study, and are forever cross-covering each other to free up days for essential courses. Some rotas allow no choice as to when holiday is taken, while others rely on the tradition of 'internal cover' by which on-call shifts that are 'missed' while on annual leave have to be paid back when the doctor returns. The MTAS debacle (a 'deeply damaging episode for British medicine' according to the man who led an independent enquiry into it, and one that I was fortunate to avoid) resulted in doctors leaving the country and the profession. Many complaints could be directed at administrative and academic bodies that are not part of the NHS: Modernising Medical Careers (MMC), Deaneries, the Royal Colleges or Medical Education England (MEE) - but the doctor in training who is struggling to progress cannot be expected to understand the subtle tensions that exist between these bodies, it just feels like the 'system' - the health service, the NHS.

Self-sufficiency

Doctors in training flit from employer to employer with great regularity. I think I worked for 9 trusts between qualification and consultancy. This unusual pattern of employment demands two qualities – adaptability and self-sufficiency. Adaptability is crucial, because you have to learn the ropes of a new hospital within days, sometimes hours, if your patients are not to be disadvantaged. Self sufficiency is equally important. The doctor who moves through an ever changing landscape of individual trusts seeks constant reassurance that their trajectory is correct, their educational development satisfactory, their emotional wellbeing monitored. They want to know that someone is keeping an eye on them. The system can meet these demands up to a point, but is designed to identify and assist outliers, the ones who are struggling. The majority will move forward, deal with their own problems and dig into their own resources to work through the crises they are bound to encounter…they will not be feel the warm hand of the 'system' at their back. So, when their training is complete and they find themselves reasonably happy with their lot, they will attribute their success to their own persistence and endurance. They will not feel grateful to the NHS for the help and encouragement that it gave. The pride that they feel will be personal.

Where does loyalty lie?

In a consultant interview one of the questions was "Will you work at XXXX, or for XXXX?" It was a good question, because it forced me to express the desire, in advance, to be loyal. I had not worked at the hospital and I did not yet know if it deserved such a commitment. Only a fool would have said, *"Oh, well...ask me again in six months and I'll tell you!"* On further reflection the question suggested that there should be automatic loyalty to an employer. I asked myself if I had demonstrated loyalty to my previous Trusts? Had I defended them when they were criticised? Had I made an extra effort at work in order to strengthen their reputation? The answer was no. I had whined and whinged about the conditions as much as my colleagues in the pub after work. I had brimmed with frustration when I couldn't get away for training days. My loyalty lay with my team, my mentors, perhaps with my department, but not with the institution itself. As the expiry date on my contract approached, as my ID card was automatically deactivated (sometimes a couple of days before I actually left), I recognised that I was another employee passing through. Close colleagues would say goodbye, emotions might run high (the most stressful jobs engender a 'band of brothers/sisters' feeling) but the hospital wouldn't blink an eye. The NHS wouldn't miss a beat. The day after I and my new friends left, a fresh group entered...and a smooth service was maintained.

We are loyal to people and to places. The great mobilization of energy by staff and community in Lewisham, south east London, to defend the downgrading of their local hospital, is a case in point. Loyalty is an emotional response, fed by proximity and constancy. Medical trainees are rather like journeymen of old, moving from Trust to Trust, trading their nascent expertise for a salary, and for the training that ensures ongoing growth, then moving on. Such journeymen do not develop loyalty easily.

Tangible and intangible rewards

Hasn't the NHS rewarded its staff for the demands it has made? Of course it has…senior doctors are well paid, and risk opprobrium when they moan about conditions on salaries that approach or exceed 6 figures. But money is not the issue, because the changes that are being made will not take it away - and of course, doctors working in the private sector will not be excluded from the financial benefits that its expansion may present. There are deeper, more subtle rewards for working as a doctor in the NHS, but they require us to step back and appreciate how amazing our jobs are. It is easy to forget that working within the huge, impersonal structure has allows us to pursue a vocation. It facilitates the practice of skills that we competed to acquire, and provides the protections and guarantees that come with state sponsorship. Although progress through the system feels random and unplanned, it is at least guaranteed to those who pass their exams and maintain standards. Patients trust us with their lives. Why don't these benefits engender loyalty? They do…but to the job, to the vocation. Not to the administrative structure within which we work. Perhaps we have been spoilt. Perhaps we will only notice how well we have been treated when that structure crumbles. To really appreciate that structure we need to look up and out, beyond the personal to the societal.

A higher level of concern

If the defenders of the NHS are not motivated by personal loyalty, what is it that gets them up in the morning? It must be because they are looking at it not as providers of healthcare but as sociologists. They are concerned about access, equality, disenfranchisement, the creation of two tiers… These concerns require a higher level of understanding. The problem, I feel, is that most of us are not influenced by these socio-political issues. We are relatively apolitical, we go with the flow, we allow changes to wash over us and hope that our lives will not be disturbed too much. Only social campaigners fight for others. The rest of us just get on.

The one thing that most healthcare workers would respond to is a threat to patient safety. No one can see into the future, no one knows if the gradual privatisation of the NHS will adversely affect the care that patients receive. The full NHS risk register was not published, but it is hoped that the very act of reading the warnings it contained allowed preparations to be made to minimise potential harms. Only as mistakes occur will the case against privatisation grow, but by then we will be reacting to downstream events, not reversing the cause. There are signs. Recently, NHS Direct pulled out of the 111 service for financial reasons. We have been reassured that patient care did not and will not suffer, although an undercover reporter said,

'*Halfway through the training a manager in the call centre admitted to me and the other trainees that on the weekends the service was 'unsafe' because they didn't have enough staff to handle calls.*'

Serco, a private contractor for out of hours primary care services in Cornwall,

'*falsified figures on its performance 252 times, making it look better than it was, so that serious failings in the service only came to light thanks to whistleblowers.*'

On the other hand we know that many harms were done to patients before the Health and Social Care Act came into being. The Francis report into Mid Staffs has demonstrated that all was not well with the current system. The NHS and safety are not synonymous. So I, as an individual doctor, with a small view, must accept that I am not in a position to know what is right . I am a worker. I see the decisions being made around me and I may feel comfortable or I may feel uncomfortable… but that is as far as it goes. I do not feel particularly sad to see the NHS changed. For the reasons explored above, loyalty to it is not woven into my DNA. But I do worry that the decision to take it apart was made for the wrong reasons. I worry that public representatives with vested interests voted in favour of privatization because they saw the opportunity to make profits. I worry that providers will walk away when promised returns to do not materialise. I worry that patients will be disadvantaged or put at risk… but these objections are hard to define and shrouded in uncertainty. Perhaps my middling, rather anaemic reaction to these changes is a typical one. That might explain the failure of the medical and nursing professions to rise up.

Near the end

An opaque code: the Liverpool Care Pathway and a gap in perception

The independent report into end of life care, 'MORE CARE, LESS PATHWAY: A REVIEW OF THE LIVERPOOL CARE PATHWAY' has been published. Eagerly awaited, following months of controversy (click on the category below for other posts) , the report contains a paragraph that at first sight seems somewhat trivial…but which I think holds a key to the whole problem,

The Review panel has reluctantly concluded that the term 'Liverpool Care Pathway' is most unhelpful: anxious and upset relatives cannot be expected to understand what an 'integrated care pathway' is, let alone what it has to do with Liverpool.

A 'pathway' suggests to most people a road that leading somewhere. When someone is 'put on' a pathway, it sounds like, as one carer put it, they are being placed on "a conveyor belt to death". In the context of the debate about assisted dying and euthanasia, some carers have formed the impression that "the pathway" represents a decision on the part of clinicians, in effect, to kill their dying patients, when that is clearly not the case.

[page 17]

The LCP controversy has highlighted many things, not least the prevalence of poor communication at the end of life, but the importance of the 'perception gap' between doctors and patients has not received much attention. The two are of course connected. The paragraph reproduced above is all about perception, and I will use it as a springboard from which to explore this aspect of the LCP.

When the LCP was first adopted I found it quite a challenge. This was because its implementation required *work*. Before the LCP a patient's final days would, in many cases, just happen. That is not to say that we were passive, lazy or negligent…just reactive. Doctors and nurses responded to symptoms and altered the care that was given appropriately. Families reported that their loved ones were in pain, we prescribed some morphine or a sedative. Often, because our minds had not been focussed on the possible burden or futility of ongoing medical treatments (such as antibiotics, infusions or tubes) they would continue by default.

The LCP ensured that these factors were *anticipated*, so the patient did not have to wait for pain killers or go through unnecessary interventions.

But the LCP was a 'thing' to be 'implemented'. And, like any new or different form of treatment, it required discussion. So I found myself sitting down with families who were often bleary eyed with tears or outright fatigue, to introduce a whole new concept. It felt uncomfortable - describing it, justifying it, 'selling' it, this Pathway, when the family were under the impression that their loved one's journey was nearly over. *Another* pathway, another plan, another change...

My initial thoughts about the LCP were, '*Why? We're doing it already. This just turns dying into another booklet...*' But its benefits became clear, and I will not describe all of them here. Because I saw those benefits I concluded that the work of describing and explaining it to families was worthwhile. It put them in the picture. It ensured that the ground was prepared for the adjustments that might be made around the bedside; the drip that might come down without being replaced, the blocked cannula that might be removed without being re-inserted, the feeding tube that might become coiled in mouth and taken away without being re-passed. Before the LCP such changes or omissions would have been discussed, of course, but now the *philosophy* of care, of minimising burden, was out in the open. But the work had to be done.

The work was complex. It was nothing less than a crash course in the pathophysiology of dying, the concept of treatment burden, the 'double effect' of opiates... all the while remaining sensitive to individual circumstances. Doctors are used to such conversations, but now there was another step...to encapsulate those principles of palliative care and present them in a new package, the LCP. Here it is. Strange words. As that paragraph from the report suggests...Liverpool – why?, Care – that's easy, Pathway – what? Well it's just a name...it means nothing. The important thing is what it means for your relative.

The acronym became familiar to doctors and nurses. In fact it became a shorthand for 'final days of life'. *He's on the LCP. She's for the LCP. Don't you think it's time for the LCP doctor?* Such phrases were not signs of a callous attitude, but instances of medical shorthand. Our conversations teem with them. And overnight, when junior doctors were called to see dying patients, it became common for that shorthand to become manifest. The LCP could be 'started' at 3am, unknown to the family. All it meant was, the patient is dying. It formalised the clinical impression. But was it too easy? It is quite possible that such automaticity led us to underestimate the gap in perception between us and our patients' families. What became shorthand for us became an impenetrable code to families. Codes suggest secrecy, sacerdotalism, an imbalance of power, decisions made without discussion.

But if we did the work, made the time to talk families through it, there was no problem. So what happened? It would seem that on numerous occasions the work of talking was squeezed out, while the implementation – all those adjustments, all those omissions – remained. The ground was not prepared. The code was applied, but the explanation was not given. Thus, as described on page 22 of the report,

As if caught in the midst of a perfect storm, relatives and carers would discover that a previously sentient person was now semi-comatose. They were told that, following an overnight decision by a relatively junior clinician, this patient had been 'placed on the pathway.'

This is the gap in perception. I, a doctor who is well used to seeing patients die, would interpret such a change in conscious level as the natural progression in a patient's terminal illness, and the LCP as being no more than a corollary to this, a way of organising his care… but in the eyes of his family there has been a deterioration COINCIDENT IN TIME with a NEW TREATMENT. How could any reasonable lay person not assume that the LCP had led to the deterioration? Without the work of explanation the LCP is therefore at best opaque and at worst, to some who feel vulnerable or poorly served by the very hospital in which their loved one failed to recover following an acute admission, outright sinister.

This excerpt crystallises another gap in perception, in the area of consent;

'No one explained anything to us about what would take place once the Pathway was implemented, or what would happen otherwise. We weren't given anything to read and, as far as I can remember, the issue was raised so tentatively by the doctor and nurse that at the time we were simply unaware that we had taken such an important decision.' [page 24]

The concern is echoed in one of the panel's conclusions,

From the submissions of evidence that the Review panel has received, it is clear that one of the central issues causing difficulty seems to be some misunderstanding and uncertainty over whether deciding to implement the LCP is a treatment decision that requires the patient's consent (if the person has capacity) or requires the decision to be taken in the patient's best interests (if the person lacks capacity). [page 23]

Decision. The leather-skinned, busy, functional doctor in me reacts to this. Decision? I know that the LCP was designed with nothing more than comfort and dignity in mind, elements of care that should not require shared decisions or consent. But the empathetic, reflective doctor in me accepts that because the LCP appears to represent a change in treatment, every effort must be made to carry the family along in complete and explicit agreement. There is no point harping on about whether consent or assent are legally required. If the conversation is had, if the work is done, the gap in perception will be filled with words and mutual understanding. But the work has to be done.

Why do I use the term 'work' so much? It sounds churlish and reluctant. I use it because I think we need to prioritise the role of the conversation, rather than let this seemingly soft side of medicine give way to the never-ending, ever more urgent list of hard tasks that our doctors, junior and senior, must accomplish in an average day. As the flow of acute admissions increases, as our patients' degree of frailty increases with the average age of the population, we have to come up with better ways of organising that 'work'. The report's introduction concludes with this entirely appropriate comment,

We feel strongly that if acute hospitals are to deal with dying patients – and they will – whether or not they are using the LCP – they need to treat patients, their relatives and carers with more respect. Hospitals and other institutions need to make more time available to them at any hour of the day or any day of the week. We know that hospitals are often short staffed, and that senior staff may often not be present at night, over weekends, and on Bank Holidays. This is perceived by many as one major cause of poor levels of care and communication. In order that everyone dying in the acute sector can do so with dignity, the present situation has to change.

Unless we can find the time to talk, at length, gaps in perception will persist, and our good intentions will continue to be misconstrued.

A new way of saying goodbye? (on Twitter)

Shortly after I joined Twitter he replied to something I wrote, and retweeted it. It was a thrill. His follow-up comments were insightful, incisive and justified. The exchange drew in some more established Tweeps, a few of them followed me, and I felt that I had truly joined the conversation. We followed each other. Thereafter we had the odd interaction, not many, but I tended to agree with him, and he with me. Once, when I felt demoralised after receiving some personal criticism during a controversial debate, he supported my point of view. Coming from him it felt important, and it cheered me up.

Months later I read a Tweet reporting that he had died. I was shocked because he had Tweeted just a few days before. Quite a few commented on his passing. I wrote something, although, never having known him, it was necessarily shallow. I didn't include his ID…that felt too direct. The brief eulogy was based on the impression I had formed over a matter of months, on fifteen, perhaps twenty micro-posts. But I was not indifferent, and had to say something.

Then I noticed that an automated daily round up of topics that had interested him was still being generated and posted in is Twitter account. His avatar kept popping into my timeline. Every time it appeared I felt a pang of grief. Then I saw that others who had been referenced in his updates were replying, thanking him for the mentions.

A week later, still haunted by these strange, autonomous updates, I tapped his avatar, took a last look at the hand-drawn likeness, and touched Unfollow. It felt like a disloyal act. Our peculiar, virtual relationship was over.

I have subsequently learned that he was a keen proponent of social media and a very generous man. I hope Twitter will bring me into contact with even more people like him…(it already has). I suppose an inevitable part of broadening your social and professional circle is that death will touch you more often. It's not yet clear to me how you respond to the death of a person whose thoughts you are accustomed to reading, but whom you have never actually known. Perhaps, just as Twitter provides a new way of knowing people, it demands a new way of saying goodbye.

Signals: the language of uncertainty

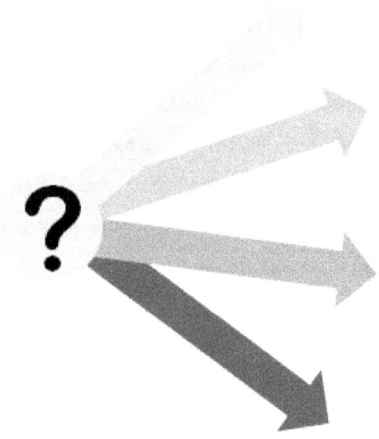

Seeing patients in the emergency department the other day, it struck me that for all my attempts to explain to patients and relatives in clear terms and recognisable words what was going on, there was one area in which communication remained unsatisfactory – prognostic uncertainty. That is, in those situations where I feel that there is a significant risk of further deterioration, and possibly death, but where it is too early to justify a full and frank discussion about ceilings of care or end of life management. After all, we typically review patients just a few hours after they have been admitted to hospital. At this stage the patient has barely had a chance to respond to the treatments that have been instituted. We have no idea what direction things are going to take.

So I ask myself – should I let the family know that their loved one could deteriorate? Of course..that's pretty obvious. But if I do that I must also broach the subject of escalation to ICU, or, if that is not to be considered appropriate, end of life care. Do I know enough about them yet to have that discussion? Perhaps I should keep my concerns to myself and wait for the patient to be reviewed again in 24 hours, by which time the trajectory of their illness, whether improving or deteriorating, will be clearer.

Personally, I believe it is more honest to explore uncertainty early on, otherwise the family may go home confident that their relative will improve, and unaware of what may happen should there be a sudden worsening in their condition. But... to introduce the concept of uncertainty and possible deterioration requires great care. Perhaps too much care, for if the language one uses is too subtle and oblique, the message can go astray.

The average ward round in an ED or acute medical unit will require one or several 'proper' sit down conversations, ideally in a room or private space, so that the doctor can discuss all eventualities. Such discussions, in my experience, are reserved for situations in which the patient appears to be dying, clearly pre-terminal, or at significant risk of suffering a cardiac arrest from which he or she will not be successfully resuscitated by CPR. The conversation with relatives will serve to explain that the short term prognosis is poor, and that CPR may not be inappropriate. But uncertainty requires a different kind of conversation, one that takes place at a less profound emotional level and does not usually cause the clinician to invoke the full panoply of communication skills. Uncertainty leads to a 'preparatory' conversation, and usually takes place at the bedside. The challenge is to balance clarity with mere suggestion, frankness with compassion and the risk of information overload with a comprehensive exploration of possible eventualities. Not only this, the messages conveyed must be understood by all of those present – the patient (often elderly), a spouse and sometimes younger members of the family. They may interpret words and signals very differently.

For example, imagine a man of 86 years who has been admitted with pneumonia. His exercise tolerance is quite poor (a hundred yards, slowly), perhaps due to chronically diseased lungs. He had a major heart attack ten years ago but got over it. The chest x-ray shows a large area of infection, but he is talking and jovial. He has received antibiotics, and requires a modest amount of oxygen.

The conversation, with the patient, his wife and a daughter, may go like this:

Doctor: It looks like a chest infection.

Patient: OK doctor. Is that all?

Doctor: Pneumonia…

Patient (recognising this word as a more grave condition): Oh!

Doctor: That's we call chest infections. It's a serious illness. Because your lungs are already a bit scarred it could go on to make you quite ill.

Wife: So it's serious then?

Doctor: It is, pneumonia is always serious. But it should respond to the antibiotics.

Patient: That's alright then…

Daughter: What do you mean by 'serious' doctor?

Doctor: It could get worse, if the infection spreads.

Daughter: And then what will you do?

Doctor: If his breathing deteriorates, and his oxygen levels fall…that would be a very worrying development.

Daughter: What would happen?

Doctor: Well…sometimes patients need more help with their breathing…

Daughter: A ventilator you mean?

Doctor: Perhaps, but we would need to ask the intensive care doctors to come and see your Dad and tell us what sort of treatments would help…

Wife: He doesn't seem that unwell at the moment doctor.

Doctor: No, he's tolerating the infection very well. It's just I think it's important that you know that pneumonia is a potentially serious illness, and patients can get worse before they get better…

Daughter: He barely sees his doctor you know. There's nothing really wrong with him.
Doctor: That is very encouraging, but the x-ray does show some signs of damage from before the infection, and that's why I'm being a bit cautious…

There are oblique phrases in here, some of which are not entirely honest of we examine the thoughts behind them:

'quite ill' – the doctor means 'critically ill'

'worrying development' meaning 'life threatening deterioration'

'patients can get worse before they get better…' meaning, in fact, 'not all who get worse will get better'

'It's just I think it's important that you know' meaning 'I really want you to take this in, I'm really worried'

'tell us what sort of treatments would help', meaning 'I can't commit to escalation to intensive care and mechanical ventilation, it's not entirely my decision…but nor do I want to engage on an escalation of care discussion at this moment…'

'cautious' meaning 'I'm very worried about your father, there's a real possibility that this infection will prove fatal'

So why use these oblique terms? Why not be clear, and say what he is actually thinking? Because the doctor has to be cautious in both directions – not too encouraging or unrealistically positive, but not too gloomy or doom-laden either. For after all, the doctor has only just met the patient and the family, and as I explained above, there is not yet enough evidence to justify an end of life type discussion.

Should the doctor discuss resuscitation? Yes, probably, but his reticence on this issue will be equally understandable. The patient is independent usually, limited yes, but with a good quality of life. And as his daughter says, there is little in the way of formally established or active co-morbidities. He may have well have chronic airways disease, but no one has told him so. There is not enough in the history to convince the consultant that he should be 'Not For Resuscitation'.

The result of all these deliberations? – neither one thing nor the other. Subtle hints, tangential phrases that may be interpreted by the daughter in one way and the patient or his wife in another. The patient may be transferred to the medical ward reassured that the antibiotics will make him better, the daughter may go home worrying about the consultant's thinly veiled pessimism, or 'caution'. And the doctor walks on to the next patient thinking he has sent out enough cautionary signals to cover all the bases. How wrong he might be.

In this article I have tried to show how challenging it is for doctors to adequately explore and communicate uncertainty in acute situations. There is little time, scarce fore-knowledge of the patient or the family, and a degree of defensiveness. The quest for improved communication continues, but here we have an example of how challenging the job can be!

Substitutes

You invite the closest relative of a critically ill patient into a private room and discuss what can be done, what can't be done, what's realistic, what's inevitable...and gain a sense of what your patient's attitude to major medical intervention might have been. You ask a question, 'What do you think they would want us to do?' You have entered into the process of eliciting a 'substituted judgment' (SJ). What would the patient have wanted if they could speak to you now, right now? If they knew what the pros and the cons were, what the risks and the benefits were, what the burdens and the rewards were, this is what they would ask you to do - Leave well alone, palliate, 'allow natural death', or go to the ends of the earth to find a cure, ventilate, dialyse, put tubes in here and tubes in there, do whatever it takes...

SJ seems to make perfect sense. It is the nearest we can get to a conversation with the patient. But what if those who are close to the patient are not, in fact, very close at all? What about patients who have become isolated, or through their lifestyles have spurned or avoided continuing contact? In such situations the opinion of a relative or a friend will be little more than guesswork. How much of their opinion will be based on supposition or reliance on their own values, or on very historical impressions that they may have gained of the patients possible desires? If the validity of that SJ is clearly challengeable, it comes back to the clinicians to start making decisions in their patient's perceived best interests. Thus the pendulum of power swings back from the patient's autonomous existence before they entered hospital to a more paternalistic, medical arena. Conscious of this, and in effort to minimise accusations of playing God, doctors are swayed by the slightest clue as revealed by the Next of Kin who attend the hospital when patients are incapacitated by illness. Great weight is placed on their words.

SJ has its critics. Looking back to its legal and philosophical underpinnings in history, it seems to derive from the 'legal fiction' created to justify the appropriation of funds from relatives who had been confined to asylums. [Louise Harmon of the Touro Law Centre](.) (New York), an evident sceptic, wrote in 1990,

'substituted judgment...has its origins in the early nineteenth-century law of lunacy. Lord Eldon crafted the legal fiction of "doing that which it is probable the lunatic himself would

have done," permitting equity courts to make gifts of the lunatic's surplus income to relatives for whom the lunatic owed no duty of support.

About twenty years ago the fiction was borrowed from the law of lunacy into the law of informed consent. There it has been used by courts to remove organs from the body of the incompetent, to sterilize him, to force medication on him, to let him wither and die, and virtually fall off the vine.'

Less trenchant critics have analysed the weaknesses of SJ in great detail, and I will summarise these later in the article. But first I will put words into the mouths of some fictional protagonists to demonstrate its frailties in a recognisable context.

oOo

She loves life you see…

A 78 year old woman, Ella Hughes, is rushed into the Emergency Department. She has suffered a heart attack and is in cardiogenic shock - her blood pressure is critically low, she is confused because her brain is not being perfused properly, and other organs are beginning to fail too. Her kidneys have shut down, her oxygen levels are low. The intensive care team have already been called to review her. It is the registrar who first speaks with her husband. Having examined the patient the registrar goes into the room with an air of pessimism. She has seen - has become persuaded - that the patient is probably dying. She introduces herself.

"Hello, I'm Sarah Jones, one of the intensive care doctors. What's your relationship to Mrs Hughes?"

"I'm her sister."

"You came into the hospital with her?"

"I was called my her warden. They've got my number."

"So where does she live?"

"Roedean Court it's called, they're warden controlled flats, you know, for..."

"Yes."

"How is she?"

"Very, very ill. She has suffered a very large heart attack. Her heart is failing as we speak. I'm sorry, but I don't think she can survive..."

"You mean she's dying?"

"I...I think so."

"There is nothing you can do?"

"There are always things that can be done, theoretically. But we have to think..."

"What 'things'? Please, tell me."

"Well..." She is disquieted. She did not expect this. She thought the relative would understand and accept that Ella was dying. "Well, there are drugs, to keep the blood pressure up...and devices...to strengthen the heart, temporarily..."

"Good. Good. So can she have those. Perhaps she will get better. The heart can recover, can't it. I had a heart attack too, five years ago...and I'm fine now."

"It's not that simple. To do those things would require taking Ella to intensive care, inserting tubes into her, a ventilator I'm sure... we have to be sure that there is reasonabe chance that these things will work, and that she would want us to do those things to her."
"Oh I'm sure she would."

"Has she spoken to you about these sort of things...about what she woud want if she was so ill."

"She has, in the past. She loves life you see. She'd do anything, go through anything, to prolong it. I know she would."

"I...I'll need to..."

"I know it's not up to me, you're the doctor, but I don't want you to give up on her. She's just come in..."

"Okay, I understand. I'll just go and talk to my consultant..."

"Good, please do. Can I go and see her?"

We'd better do it.

Dr Jones rings her consultant.

"Her sister wants everything."

"Has the patient said anything?"

"No, she's barely conscious now."

"Is she dying, now, in your opinion?"

"Well yes, but that's inevitable if we don't support her. The question is should we support her. When I saw her I assume not, she was so sick, but the ED staff have put her on CPAP, started some Dobutamine, she looks better."

"So you may have made the wrong call. The ED have done the right thing to keep her going. What about the cardiologists, can they cath her? That's what she needs isn't it.?"
"No. Too unstable. They think she needs a balloon pump for 24 hours, then review."
"We'd better do it."

She hardly sees her!

Ella is transferred to ICU, sedated, ventilated, central lines inserted, haemofiltration catheter, and a balloon via her femoral artery into the aorta. She remains unstable. She remains silent. Sarah Jones is back on the unit 24 hours later. She sees a man enter the unit to visit Ella.

"Hello. Are you one of Ella's relatives?"

"I'm her husband. Tony Hughes."

"Oh...I thought..."

"We were divorced many years ago. But when I heard that she was so ill I decided to come in."

"Her sister rang you?"

"Her sister. What, Dorothy? No, our daughter called me. Has Dorothy been here then?"
"She was with her when Ella came in. She is down as Ella's nexy of kin actually, so we have been talking to her quite alot."

Mr Hughes looks uncomfortable and unhappy.

"What's the matter."

"Dorothy doesn't know her at all! She hardly sees her!"

Don't let anyone keep me going like that

Sarah speaks with the consultant in charge of the unit - not the one who was on call on the day of her admission.

"I spoke to her for twenty minutes, she convinced me that Mrs Hughes would want aggressive treatment. Now I find out she barely knows her sister. Lives three miles away but sees her once a year or something."

"But it's all we've got to go on isn't it? It's the closest we've got."

"I think the husband knows her better."

"And what does he say?"

"That she'd hate to be as she is now, connected to machine et cetera. He bases that on the fact that the were married when Ella own father died of cancer and Ella said something along the lines of 'don't let anyone keep me going like that.' But this was over a quarter of a century ago."

"How did the sister get such a different impression?"

"She bases that on the fact that Ella was always so vivacious, energetic and positive. She lives abroad, that's where she met her husband, and travelled extensively. She was a prominent feminist, a journalist in the seventies, then developed depression."

"You know all about her."

"Her husband was very helpful."

Another day. There is no improvement. The intensivists and the cardiologists discuss her prospects at the end of the bed.

"The echo shows her aortic valve is tight. The angio we did yesterday wasn't too bad. What she needs is a new aortic valve, a transcatheter aortic valve implantation, a TAVI. It's not entirely out of the question, if she remains like this and no worse."
"She's on multiple organ support. We were coming to the conclusion that this is an unsurvivable situation."

"Perhaps it is. Perhaps not. What do the family say?"

"There's a...difference of opinion."

"Strong either way?"

"Not unreasonably so. Neither relative can tell us with any confidence how far Mrs Hughes would want to go."

"Well I can make an estimate, say 30-40%, that she will survive. There are other risks of course, like stroke. We'll leave to option out there. I'm happy to speak to the family myself, if you think that would help. Who is the next of kin?"

"On paper...her sister."

"And she's..."

"Pro everything."

I felt like I was responsible

Her sister returns home, and phones a close friend.

"It was strange. I felt like I was responsible. They asked me what they should do. Well, they seemed to need my opinion, and what could I say? It sounded like they were giving up on her already. I couldn't let them do that without challenging them. We haven't been close since we were teenagers, it's probably my fault, I wasn't there for her when she developed depression, and she didn't come to me when she was getting divorced. I've always felt guilty about that. But now, if there's sometying I can do for her I'm going to do it, and if that means fighting her corner while the doctors try to turn away I'm going to do it!"

Her ex-husband phones their daughter.

"Hello Mary. She's bad. They're doing their best but it's a terrible sight. Tubes everywhere, totally sedated. They seem to be unsure about what to do next, whether to send her to London for an operation or let nature take its course. Your aunt seemed to think she'd want to go through anything to last a bit longer, but I'm not at all sure."

"Is it up to us then?"

"I don't think so. But if it's a borderline situation, medically, perhaps what we say will make a difference. They asked your aunt about resuscitation I think, and she said they should give her mouth to mouth and all that! I tried to let them know that I thought that was going too far. I mean, I know I haven't spoken to your mother for a few years now, but would she really want that?"

"We've never really talked about these things."

"Well we did, when her father was dying. She was very forthright."

"Then you should tell the doctors."

"But that was years ago, and a completely different situation. They won't want to hear all about that."

"I'll go in and speak to them. Will this operation they're talking about work?"

"They're not sure. It's risky."

On the ICU

"Day 4. Are we getting anywhere?"

"Not really. Inotropes are down, but she's still in multiple organ failure."

"I think we should pull out. She's not going to survive this."

"Her sister won't be happy."

"None of us are happy. It's a sad, terribly sad situation. But if we genuinely believe that all this is becoming futile it's all rather academic. Nothing is going to make a difference. The TAVI is pie in the sky, I've been there before, the chance of her getting accepted and transferred is so small." Turning to the nurse, "Can you ask the next of kin in this afternoon, I'll speak with them. It's a sister isn't it?"

oOo

The case of Karen Quinlan

The relevance of substituted judgment in medical ethics was first explored properly in law during the case of Karen Quinlan, a 21 year old woman from Pennsylvania who sustained severe brain damage a 15-20 minute respiratory arrest attributed to an accidental overdose of diazepam, dextropropoxyphene (an opioid that used to be an ingredient of Coproxamol in the

UK) and alcohol. Karen had been dieting to fit into a party dress, had barely eaten for two days, and weighed 52kg. She ended up in a persistent vegetative state. Her father, a Catholic, argued in that she would not want to remain alive in such a state, and the judge allowed her doctors to disconnect the respirator. She survived, breathing unaided, for another 9 years, and eventually succumbed to pneumonia.

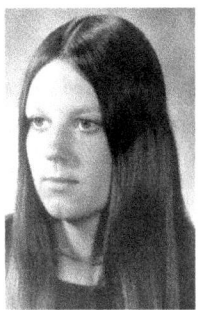

Karen Quinlan, image from Wikipedia

After much discourse, which included reviewing '...the reasoning expressed by Pope Pius XII in his "allocutio" (address) to anesthesiologists on November 24, 1957', the judge wrote:

Our affirmation of Karen's independent right of choice, however, would ordinarily be based upon her competency to assert it. The sad truth, however, is that she is grossly incompetent and we cannot discern her supposed choice based on the testimony of her previous conversations with friends, where such testimony is without sufficient probative weight.

Nevertheless we have concluded that Karen's right of privacy [which is taken to mean 'the right to be left alone', or not to be subjected to 'extraordinary means' to preserve life in this context] *may be asserted on her behalf by her guardian under the peculiar circumstances here present.*

If a putative decision by Karen to permit this non-cognitive, vegetative existence to terminate by natural forces is regarded as a valuable incident of her right of privacy, as we believe it to be, then it should not be discarded solely on the basis that her condition prevents her conscious exercise of the choice.

The only practical way to prevent destruction of the right is to permit the guardian and family of Karen to render their best judgment, subject to the qualifications hereinafter stated, as to whether she would exercise it in these circumstances.

If their conclusion is in the affirmative this decision should be accepted by a society the overwhelming majority of whose members would, we think, in similar circumstances, exercise such a choice in the same way for themselves or for those closest to them.

It is for this reason that we determine that Karen's right of privacy may be asserted in her behalf, in this respect, by her guardian and family under the particular circumstances.

It is quite affecting to read this in the original judgment (linked above) – the legal underpinning (in the United States at any rate) for an essential part of daily medical practice!

Inconsistencies and ignorance

Criticisms of substituted judgment are articulated very well in a 2008 paper by Alexia Torke, G. Caleb Alexander and John Lantos, 'Substituted Judgment: The Limitations of Autonomy in Surrogate Decision Making.' They firstly explain how,

'The philosophical appeal of this standard is that it supports the patient's autonomy by leading us to the decision that the patient would have wanted.'

But the essential problems are, according the authors, threefold;

- *Inconsistency*: studies show that peoples' opinions about what they would want change over time,

'In one study over half of patients who initially said yes to a series of medical procedures changed their minds over two years. Furthermore, mind-changing is not random. Individuals who fill out an advanced directive are less likely to change their wishes than those who do not. Thus, the patients who most need substituted judgment, because they lack a living will, are the ones for whom it is least likely to be accurate.'

- *Inaccuracy*; relatives are not good at understanding what patients 'would have wanted'

'A recent meta-analysis of surrogate predictions found that surrogates are correct about 68% of the time'

- *Patient preference*; patients may not actually want their presumed former opinions to be a major factor in decision making at such times

'…there has been extensive research examining whether patients really want their prior wishes to be the sole basis for decisions made on their behalf. This research reveals that the majority of patients prefer that family members or physicians have input into the decisions. In these studies, as in the ones examining the stability of patients' preferences, the patients who were most likely to want their wishes to prevail were the ones who more often wrote advanced directives.'

There are other concerns, such as the subconscious tendency of relatives to 'project' their own beliefs. And what of the overwhelming nature of the task that is presented to relatives? The rules of this strange, imaginary exercise are unknown. As Linus Brostrom writes about this problem of 'underdetermination' (in his thesis 'The Substituted Judgment standard: studies on the ethics of surrogate decision making'),

All it assumes about it is that the patient is "competent". But, first, it does not clarify how competent the patient should be imagined to be. And second, neither does it clarify any other aspect of the patient's hypothesized condition, such as the patient's (hypothetical) beliefs, values, commitments, emotions, mood, or the external circumstances surrounding the decision. Depending on how the scenario is described in these regards, this could presumably have consequences for what the patient would have decided.

Confused? Imagine being asked to make sense of it in the ED.

The Mental Capacity Act - why worry?

Keen students of the UK's Mental Capacity Act will know that decisions made by medical staff, or the courts should it come to that, do *not* depend on SJ. So why the worry? Although a rigorous and subtle approach to determining the patient's 'best interests' is required, I am sure most clinicians will recognise the process of trying to work out what the patient 'would have wanted'. It comes naturally as part of caring for a patient, as an exercise in re-creating them as whole, competent, communicating persona. What is more, legal authorities do tend to accept that act of exploring what a patient felt about certain circumstances (eg. terminal illness, or resuscitation) overlaps, to some extent, with SJ. For where do we find that evidence of prior thoughts and feelings but in those closest to the patient?

Antal Szerletics writes in a useful review, 'Best interests decision-making under the Mental Capacity Act',

'The Court also makes it clear that the English notion of objective best interests cannot be equated with the substituted judgment approach as adopted in the United States but the views and the personality of P will necessarily form part of the best interests assessment.'

The author then reproduces part of a judgement, concerning a patient, P:

- *P's wishes and feelings will always be a significant factor to which the court must pay close regard.*
- *Secondly, the weight to be attached to P's wishes and feelings will always be case-specific and fact-specific. In some cases, in some situations, they may carry much, even, on occasions, preponderant, weight. In other cases, in other situations, and even where the circumstances may have some superficial similarity, they may carry very little weight. One cannot, as it were, attribute any particular a priori weight or importance to P's wishes and feelings; it all depends, it must depend, upon the individual circumstances of the particular case.*

It sounds very much like to SJ to me, as a non-lawyer.

Life Story

Alexander Torke and colleagues propose an alternative: referring to and using the patient's 'life story'. Thus,

'Surrogates consider the life story of the patient and make decisions that seem consistent in light of the patient's previous choices and experiences. A narrative approach acknowledges that when individuals lose decision making capacity, they can no longer control their health care decisions. This loss of control, however, does not mean a loss of individuality or dignity. Such basic aspects of a human being can be carried on by loved ones who make decisions for the individual that are consistent with his or her own life choices. By such an approach, surrogates do not try to predict the actual choices that an incapacitated loved one would have made, as they would under substituted judgment. ***Instead, they make decisions that consider the individual's interests and values in the context of their current situation.****'*

This simple approach is very appealing, and, I would argue, perfectly natural. I would imagine that most relatives, when asked what they think the patient would want, actually go through a similar thought process anyway. To do this requires knowledge and imagination – it is a form of extrapolation, such that the result in based in reality but can stand unsupported without true evidence. Guesswork perhaps, but inspired by proximity and emotional insight, and facilitated by a sensitive health care professional who can supply a medically accurate context.

This approach has been accepted by the American Medical Association, which writes,

'...much empirical research indicates a low correlation between proxies' decisions and what patients would have decided in hypothetical situations. Because there is no direct deductive relationship between values and a particular choice, or between previous decisions and current positions, the surrogate is often left to make an approximation of what the patient would have wanted. At best, substitute decision making requires great imaginative effort to process a patient's web of values, preferences, and medical judgments.

Rather than attempt to predict what the patient would say about treatment preferences, the patient's ***life story*** *is considered, and a particular option is evaluated in terms of its "fit" with the elements of the patient's life story. This narrative model rests on the idea that*

individuals create an identity for themselves through their life story and it is through this narrative that persons conceptualize themselves. Thus, the physician and the surrogate have a prima facie moral obligation to continue the story in a manner that is meaningful and consistent with the patient's self-conception. It is possible that more than one choice is compatible with the patient's self-conception.'

So, it seems the principle of SJ, on which we rely to guide our decisions, is flawed. Should we be worried. I don't think so. Why? Because I don't think we *do* rely on SJ. How many of us have asked a relative or loved one to actually make a decision? Few, I would say. The way we deal with such situations is to talk, to feel our way into the mind of the patient through the Next of Kin, to gain a sense of what they would be happy with and how much suffering, risk or chance they might accept in proportion to the possible gains. I think that most of us talk, converse, share, learn and, finally, approach consensus by tactfully and empathetically filling the gap in the 'life story' that is described to us. Having read the research, criticisms, studies and articles, I fail to recognise in my own practice, or that of my past trainers or current colleagues, the exercise of pure SJ. The good doctors begin to write that life story in their head as soon as they meet the relatives. It is an art and a skill that those who meet hundreds of patients per year develop naturally.

oOo

The final thoughts of Ella Hughes

"What did I really want? I can think it, but I can't tell you, not from where I lie. Suffice to say, it has hurt. I have suffered. For a while I thought it might be worth it. I caught a few words from the heart doctor…he was talking about some operation. I was hopeful. Then it all went silent. No more talk about a new valve. And that was my last chance, I think. Now I am going downhill. I believe they have given up. I don't mind, because I know I am dying. It was obvious to me from the moment I collapsed. But I wish they could have made up their minds earlier, and not prevaricated. If there was nothing that could be done, fine…don't do it. But they talked to my sister. My sister! At least Tony knew me for what I am - a pragmatist. He would have told them the truth about me. Do only what is useful, don't do anything just for the sake of it, for some idealistic 'life at all costs' ideology. I don't suppose they do that anyway nowadays…but he'll have told them. That's been the story of my whole life..pragmatic, no frills, no waste, no fuss…'

*

I am very grateful to Katherine Sleeman, palliative care registrar and clinical lecturer at Kings College London (Twitter: @kesleeman) who made some very helpful comments regarding the differences between US and UK law when this post was first published.

www.ingramcontent.com/pod-product-compliance
Lightning Source LLC
Chambersburg PA
CBHW051713170526
45167CB00002B/643